Foreword by Diabetes UK

Carbohydrate counting is an important part of diabetes management, especially for people with Type 1 diabetes.

Carbs & Cals: A visual guide to Carbohydrate & Calorie Counting is a great tool for those people with diabetes who count carbohydrates as part of the management of their condition. This easy to use visual reference guide allows you to compare what is on your plate with the picture in the book, to find out the amount of carbohydrate and the calories the food you are eating contains. Knowing how many calories in a portion of the food you are eating is also really helpful information for people who are trying to lose weight, and may let you know that you need to eat a smaller portion or opt for something a little healthier.

Having all of this information at your fingertips, in an easy to understand format, will help to give you greater control over your diabetes and also give you the information you need to help you make healthier choices at meal times. Whatever your goals we are sure that you will find *Carbs & Cals* a great help in achieving them.

Simon O'Neill
Director of Care, Information
& Advocacy Services
Diabetes UK

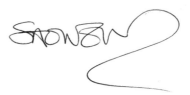

DIABETES UK
CARE. CONNECT. CAMPAIGN.

Introduction

Welcome to Carbs & Cals. This is a unique book; unlike most books, there are lots of pictures and few words.

This book has been produced with two main purposes in mind; first and foremost it provides a fantastic resource for anyone with diabetes who is carbohydrate counting or thinking of learning to carbohydrate count. Secondly, for anyone who is trying to lose weight by counting calories or needs advice on portion control, it is a great visual reference to hundreds of different food items and drinks. For the first time, it gives you the ability to see photos of the portions you could choose, and how many calories you could save by making reductions in portion sizes or choosing lower calorie alternatives.

We have included a large selection of popular food items, meals and drinks. However, as this is primarily a carbohydrate counting book, foods with no or minimal carbohydrate content have not been included. These include meat and fish steaks, as well as eggs, cheese, oils, spreads, and some vegetables.

We hope you enjoy the book and that it makes the process of carbohydrate counting easier to understand.

What is carbohydrate?

There are three main nutrients in the diet: fat, protein and carbohydrate.

Carbohydrate foods provide the body with its main energy source, which is glucose. Carbohydrate is broken down by the body into glucose, which then enters the blood. The rate at which carbohydrate is broken down depends on the type of carbohydrate eaten; this is known as the glycaemic index (GI). For example, foods with a high GI are broken down quickly causing a quick increase in blood glucose, whereas foods with a low GI are broken down slowly giving a more gradual increase.

For people managing their diabetes with insulin, it is useful to have an understanding of the speed at which blood glucose may rise after certain meals or snacks. This can help you to predict your blood glucose level after eating or drinking. If you are adjusting insulin, speak to your diabetes team about this in more detail.

One of the main drawbacks of GI is that it does not take into account the other nutrients in the meal (e.g. protein and fat content), which can slow the absorption of glucose into the blood stream. It also fails to take into account the amount of carbohydrate in the meal, which is a much better predictor of blood glucose response. For people with diabetes, it is therefore important that they have an understanding of the total carbohydrate content of the food and drink they are consuming.

The table on the next page shows the main types of food that we eat that contain carbohydrate.

Food Group	Examples	Role
Starchy Foods	Bread, potato, rice, pasta, noodles, breakfast cereal, pastry, yam, cassava, and grains e.g. couscous	Provides fibre, especially wholegrain varieties. Also an important source of calcium, iron and B vitamins
Fruit & Vegetables	All types of fruit contain carbohydrate in the form of natural fruit sugar (fructose). Vegetables vary in the amount of carbohydrate they contain but are generally slowly absorbed and do not need to be counted	A great source of vitamins, minerals and fibre
Dairy Foods	Milk, yoghurt, and ice cream all contain milk sugar (lactose)	Provides an important source of calcium, vitamins A and B12. Also a source of protein
Sugary Foods & Drinks	Sugar, jam, marmalade, honey, soft drinks, sweets, cakes, biscuits and chocolates	No nutritional benefits other than providing additional calories

How much carbohydrate should I eat each day?

The amount of carbohydrate we should eat in a day varies from person to person depending on your activity levels, gender, age and weight. It is estimated that we should get around 50% of our energy from carbohydrate. No more than 35% should come from fat and around 10-20% should be from protein.

There are 5 main food groups. The Eatwell Plate shows how much of what you eat and drink should come from each food group. This includes everything you eat and drink during the day, including snacks. Try to eat plenty of fruit and vegetables, include bread, rice, potatoes, pasta and other starchy foods at each meal (choose wholegrain varieties whenever you can), some milk and dairy foods, some meat, fish, eggs, beans and other non-dairy sources of protein, and just a small amount of food and drinks that are high in fat and/or sugar.

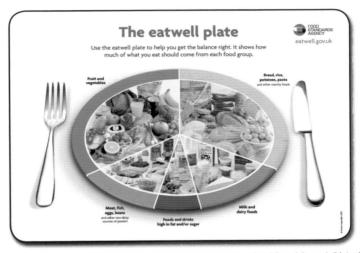

Diabetes UK is currently reviewing the recommendation for carbohydrate intake and it is possible that scientific evidence may result in the value being amended in the future.

The following table shows the amount of carbohydrate per day for different calorie intakes based on it providing 50% of energy. A registered dietitian can help you to work out how many calories per day you should aim for.

Calories	Carbohydrate per day (based on 50% of calories)
1500 kcal	190g
2000 kcal	250g
2500 kcal	315g
3000 kcal	375g

Diabetes and carbohydrate counting

Carbohydrate counting for people with diabetes is not a new concept; it has been around for over 50 years. However, in recent years it has been incorporated more and more into the education and management of Type 1, Type 2 and diabetes in pregnancy.

If you are starting out with carbohydrate counting, there are three main steps:

1. Learning about the concept of carbohydrate counting and how to estimate the amount of carbohydrate in foods and drinks.

2. Understanding the relationships between food, diabetes medications, physical activity, and blood glucose level, and how to manage these factors.

3. If you have Type 1 diabetes and are using multiple daily injections or an insulin pump, learning how to match quick-acting insulin to carbohydrate, using carbohydrate-to-insulin ratios.

Learning to estimate the amount of carbohydrate can be hard work and very time-consuming. Eating out, take-away meals and dinner with friends can be especially challenging, as it is difficult to know what ingredients have been used and you may be eating foods that are not part of your everyday diet. But with time and the right support, for most people with diabetes this becomes second nature.

Carbohydrate from the food and drink we consume is broken down into glucose. This glucose is then transferred into the blood and from there it is carried into cells of the body by the hormone insulin. The amount of insulin required is directly related to the total amount of carbohydrate being eaten.

Due to the development of newer insulin, adjusting the dose of insulin to the specific amount of carbohydrate eaten has become possible. By adjusting insulin it is possible to have greater flexibility of food choice, reduced risk of hypoglycaemia and improved blood glucose control.

For people on multiple daily injections of insulin (basal bolus) or insulin pumps, knowing the amount of carbohydrate is important to make decisions about the amount of insulin to use. Many people on two injections a day find it useful to count carbohydrate in order to keep to consistent amounts at meals from day-to-day.

In the UK, people with diabetes who are learning about carbohydrate counting are usually taught to take an amount of insulin based on each 10g of carbohydrate they eat. For example, many people are started on 1 unit of quick-acting insulin for every 10g of carbohydrate they consume. This rate will vary from person to person and can also vary at different times of the day. Your diabetes team can help to advise you on this. Please consult your diabetes team for more information.

Learning how to adjust insulin and count carbohydrate can be complex. This book is not designed to teach you how to adjust your insulin; it is important that you have the support of appropriately-trained healthcare professionals such as a diabetes specialist nurse and diabetes specialist dietitian. Many areas of the UK now offer structured education courses such as BERTIE and DAFNE for Type 1 diabetes, and X-PERT and DESMOND for Type 2 diabetes. Ask your diabetes team what is available in your area.

It is important to note that certain foods which are broken down into glucose very slowly may not require insulin or may require a reduced dose. This includes foods such as pearl barley, peas, beans and lentils, some vegetables including sweetcorn, squash/pumpkin and parsnips. It is important that you speak with your diabetes team about whether you may need to take insulin for these foods as it varies from person to person and on the amount eaten.

Carbohydrate in alcoholic drinks

Carbohydrate values of alcoholic drinks have been included in this book. These have been included as a reference only as generally it is not recommended to take additional insulin for the carbohydrate found in some alcoholic drinks. **Extreme caution should be taken when giving additional units of insulin with alcohol as you are more prone to hypoglycaemia (low blood glucose).** Speak to your diabetes team about this in more detail.

What are calories?

Calories are units of energy. They are used to measure the amount of energy in food and drinks. This energy comes from the nutrients carbohydrate, fat, protein and alcohol. Each of these nutrients contain a different number of calories per gram:

1g Carbohydrate	=	4 calories
1g Fat	=	9 calories
1g Protein	=	4 calories
1g Alcohol	=	7 calories

As seen above, fat has the most calories per gram. This is why if you eat a lot of foods that are high in fat, you are likely to consume more calories and gain more weight.

People often associate carbohydrate with being 'fattening'. However as you can see, carbohydrate contains less than half the calories of fat, and the same calories per gram as protein. Adding extra fat to the carbohydrate food (e.g. adding butter to a jacket potato, or frying) increases the calorie content.

How many calories should I eat each day?
The amount of calories a person should eat or drink depends on a number of different factors. These include age, gender, physical activity levels and whether or not you are trying to lose, maintain or gain weight. It is possible to get a more accurate idea of your calorie needs by speaking to a registered dietitian. The guideline daily amount (GDA) for calories for a female is 2000, and 2500 for men. These figures are based on an average person. Sometimes GDAs are labelled 'for adults' - these figures are based on the GDA for women to encourage people who need less energy to consume fewer calories.

Why count calories?
If you are trying to lose weight, it is useful to have an understanding of the calories in the food and drink you consume and how this compares to your requirements. It is also useful to have a realistic expectation of how many calories to cut down on and what weight loss to expect.

Studies have shown that in order to lose 0.5kg (1lb) of body weight over a week, you need to reduce calories by around 500 per day (3500 per week). This reduction could be by diet alone, or by a combination of diet and increased physical activity. By eating a smaller portion or going for a healthier snack, this should be more achievable. Below is an example of how you could save 336 calories by choosing a healthier snack:

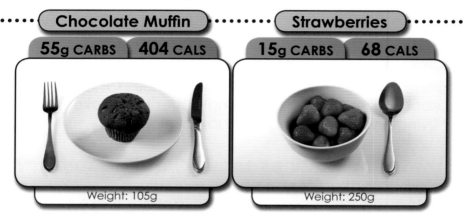

Chocolate Muffin

55g CARBS   **404** CALS

Weight: 105g

Strawberries

15g CARBS   **68** CALS

Weight: 250g

Advice on losing weight

If you are trying to lose weight it is important to follow a balanced diet, including foods from all groups. You may wish to speak to a healthcare professional such as your GP, practice nurse or registered dietitian. If you have diabetes and take diabetes medication and/or insulin, weight loss may require a change in medication; it is best to seek medical advice first.

The British Dietetic Association (BDA) has developed a website (www.bdaweightwise.com) containing lots of useful hints and tips on losing weight. Diabetes UK (www.diabetes.org.uk) also has advice on weight loss, shopping tips and recipe ideas. Commercial slimming clubs such as Weight Watchers and Rosemary Conley can also provide support.

How to use this book

Carbs & Cals has been written with complete practicality in mind. The process of using the book is as follows:

1. Prepare your meal, drink or snack as normal.
2. Find the meal, drink or snack in the book.
3. Choose the portion photo that is closest to your own.
4. If you are carb counting, use the value in green above that photo, and if you are calorie counting, use the value in blue above that photo.
5. Add up the carb or calorie values for the different food components to give the totals for your meal.

All foods are displayed on one of the following dishes:

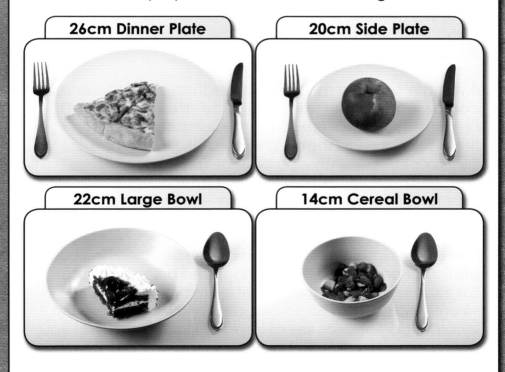

26cm Dinner Plate	20cm Side Plate

22cm Large Bowl	14cm Cereal Bowl

Each picture displays either a knife & fork, or a dessert spoon to help with scale. It may be a good idea to measure your own crockery to see how the size of your plates and bowls compares with the ones in the pictures, and possibly choose plates and bowls of a similar size to the ones shown to make it as easy as possible.

Foods are arranged in alphabetical sections of Biscuits & Crackers; Bread; Breakfast; Cakes & Bakery; Desserts; Drinks; Fruit; Meals; Meal Accompaniments; Meat & Fish Products; Potatoes; Rice, Pasta & Grains; Snacks & Confectionery; Take-away Food; and Vegetables & Pulses. The different sections are coloured so it's easy to find the food or drink you are looking for.

Please note that items in the Take-away Food section may be foods that people make at home, but for the purpose of this book the foods used and the values calculated were from take-away versions.

If you are eating a meal with more than one food or drink containing carbohydrate (e.g. roast dinner, or cooked breakfast), you will need to find each component in the book and add them up separately. For example, your roast dinner may comprise of Yorkshire puddings from p152, stuffing from p152, roast potatoes from p171, parsnips from p231, and cranberry sauce from p153.

Each food has between 1 and 6 portion examples, so you can easily judge the carbohydrate and calories in your particular portion just by looking at the different photos. For example, a digestive biscuit is always the same size, so only 1 photo has been included. However, there are 6 different portion pictures of lasagne included so that you can choose the portion that is closest to the portion on your plate.

The carbohydrate value is always in a large green tab, and the calorie value is in a large blue tab, so it's easy to see the values you are looking for.

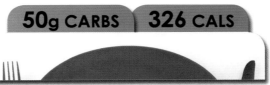

50g CARBS **326 CALS**

The weight of each portion is stated below each photo, just in case you want to double-check the weight of your own portion. **This is always the cooked / prepared weight.**

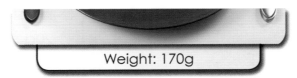

Weight: 170g

For foods that you are likely to have several of, there is a table with the carbs and cals for 1, 2, 3 and 4 pieces, to make it even easier for you to add up.

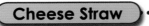

Cheese Straw

3g CARBS **38 CALS**

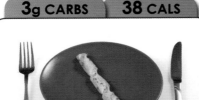

	CARBS	CALS
2x	6g	76
3x	9g	114
4x	12g	152
Weight: 7g		

Potato Waffle

15g CARBS **119 CALS**

	CARBS	CALS
2x	30g	238
3x	45g	357
4x	60g	476
Weight: 49g		

Bourbon Cream

8g CARBS   **58 CALS**

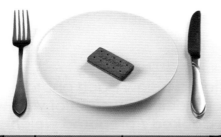

	CARBS	CALS
2x	16g	116
3x	24g	174
4x	32g	232
Weight: 12g		

Chocolate Digestive

10g CARBS   **74 CALS**

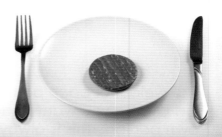

	CARBS	CALS
2x	20g	148
3x	30g	222
4x	40g	296
Weight: 15g		

Chocolate Chip Cookie

7g CARBS   **47 CALS**

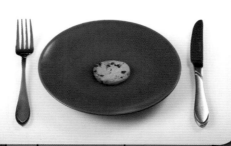

	CARBS	CALS
2x	14g	94
3x	21g	141
4x	28g	188
Weight: 10g		

48g CARBS   **351 CALS**

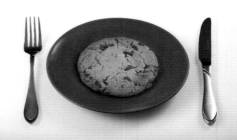

	CARBS	CALS
2x	96g	702
3x	144g	1053
4x	192g	1404
Weight: 74g		

Chocolate Oat Biscuit

12g CARBS   **91 CALS**

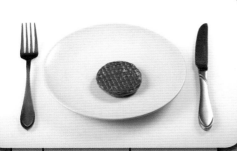

	CARBS	CALS
2x	24g	182
3x	36g	273
4x	48g	364
Weight: 19g		

Custard Cream

8g CARBS   **61 CALS**

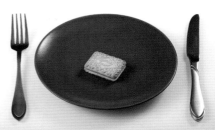

	CARBS	CALS
2x	16g	122
3x	24g	183
4x	32g	244
Weight: 12g		

Digestive

10g CARBS   **70 CALS**

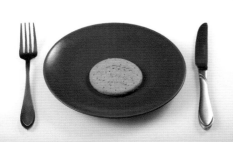

	CARBS	CALS
2x	20g	140
3x	30g	210
4x	40g	280
Weight: 15g		

Fig Roll

15g CARBS   **79 CALS**

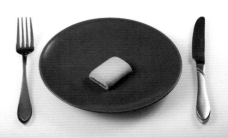

	CARBS	CALS
2x	30g	158
3x	45g	237
4x	60g	316
Weight: 21g		

Ginger Biscuit

8g CARBS   **44 CALS**

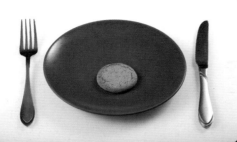

	CARBS	CALS
2x	16g	88
3x	24g	132
4x	32g	176
Weight: 10g		

Gingerbread Man

38g CARBS   **222 CALS**

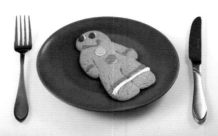

	CARBS	CALS
2x	76g	444
3x	114g	666
4x	152g	888
Weight: 58g		

Iced Ring

5g CARBS   **28 CALS**

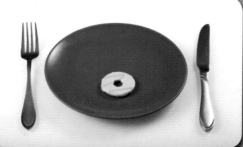

	CARBS	CALS
2x	10g	56
3x	15g	84
4x	20g	112
Weight: 6g		

Jaffa Cake

10g CARBS   **49 CALS**

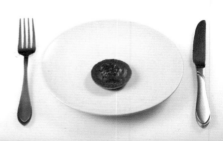

	CARBS	CALS
2x	20g	98
3x	30g	147
4x	40g	196
Weight: 13g		

Jam Ring

13g CARBS   **79 CALS**

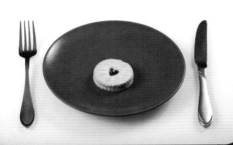

	CARBS	CALS
2x	26g	158
3x	39g	237
4x	52g	316
Weight: 18g		

Malted Milk

5g CARBS   **39 CALS**

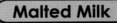
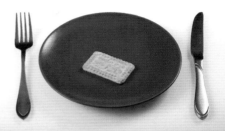

	CARBS	CALS
2x	10g	78
3x	15g	117
4x	20g	156
Weight: 8g		

Nice

5g CARBS   **39 CALS**

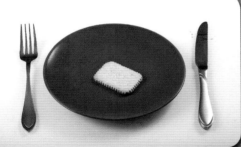

	CARBS	CALS
2x	10g	78
3x	15g	117
4x	20g	156
Weight: 8g		

Oat Biscuit

10g CARBS   **75 CALS**

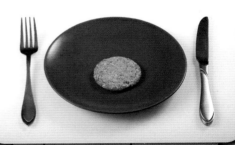

	CARBS	CALS
2x	20g	150
3x	30g	225
4x	40g	300
Weight: 16g		

20cm Side Plate

Pink Wafer

6g CARBS **48 CALS**

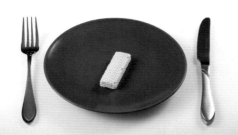

	CARBS	CALS
2x	12g	96
3x	18g	144
4x	24g	192
Weight: 9g		

Rich Tea

5g CARBS **32 CALS**

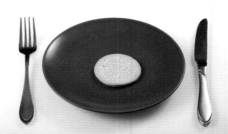

	CARBS	CALS
2x	10g	64
3x	15g	96
4x	20g	128
Weight: 7g		

Shortbread Finger

10g CARBS **81 CALS**

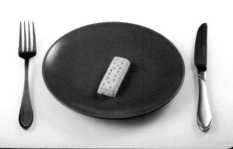

	CARBS	CALS
2x	20g	162
3x	30g	243
4x	40g	324
Weight: 16g		

Shortcake

7g CARBS **49 CALS**

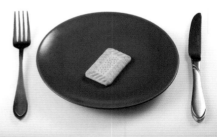

	CARBS	CALS
2x	14g	98
3x	21g	147
4x	28g	196
Weight: 10g		

Breadstick

4g CARBS   **20 CALS**

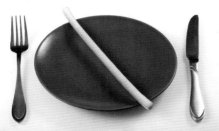

	CARBS	CALS
2x	8g	40
3x	12g	60
4x	16g	80
Weight: 5g		

Cheddar

3g CARBS   **26 CALS**

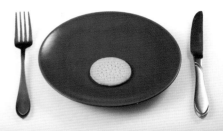

	CARBS	CALS
2x	6g	52
3x	9g	78
4x	12g	104
Weight: 5g		

Cheese Straw

3g CARBS   **38 CALS**

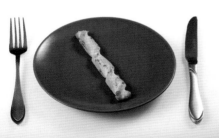

	CARBS	CALS
2x	6g	76
3x	9g	114
4x	12g	152
Weight: 7g		

Cream Cracker

5g CARBS   **33 CALS**

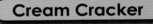

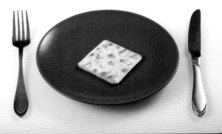

	CARBS	CALS
2x	10g	66
3x	15g	99
4x	20g	132
Weight: 8g		

Crispbread

4g CARBS	18 CALS

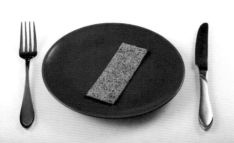

	CARBS	CALS
2x	8g	36
3x	12g	54
4x	16g	72
Weight: 6g (thin)		

8g CARBS	35 CALS

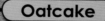

	CARBS	CALS
2x	16g	70
3x	24g	105
4x	32g	140
Weight: 11g		

Digestive (savoury)

9g CARBS	61 CALS

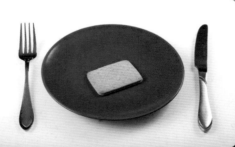

	CARBS	CALS
2x	18g	122
3x	27g	183
4x	36g	244
Weight: 13g		

Oatcake

6g CARBS	41 CALS

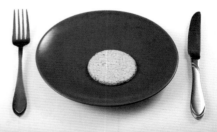

	CARBS	CALS
2x	12g	82
3x	18g	123
4x	24g	164
Weight: 10g		

Puffed Cracker

5g CARBS   **48 CALS**

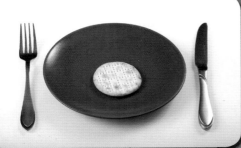

	CARBS	CALS
2x	10g	96
3x	15g	144
4x	20g	192
Weight: 9g		

Rice Cake

6g CARBS   **30 CALS**

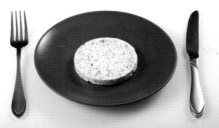

	CARBS	CALS
2x	12g	60
3x	18g	90
4x	24g	120
Weight: 8g		

Water Biscuit

5g CARBS   **26 CALS**

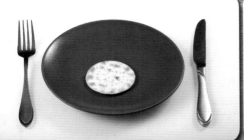

	CARBS	CALS
2x	10g	52
3x	15g	78
4x	20g	104
Weight: 6g		

Wholegrain Cracker

6g CARBS   **33 CALS**

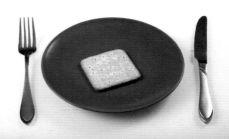

	CARBS	CALS
2x	12g	66
3x	18g	99
4x	24g	132
Weight: 8g		

Sliced Bread (granary)

5g CARBS	**26 CALS**

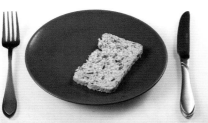

Weight: 11g (thin slice)

10g CARBS	**52 CALS**

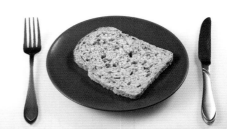

Weight: 22g (thin slice)

16g CARBS	**78 CALS**

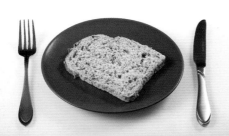

Weight: 33g (medium slice)

21g CARBS	**104 CALS**

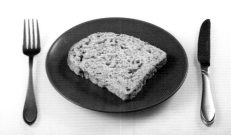

Weight: 44g (thick slice)

30g CARBS	**152 CALS**

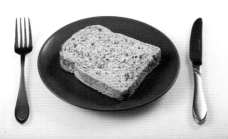

Weight: 64g (extra thick slice)

41g CARBS	**204 CALS**

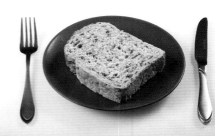

Weight: 86g

Sliced Bread (white)

5g CARBS   **24 CALS**

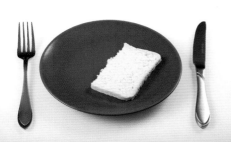

Weight: 11g (thin slice)

10g CARBS   **48 CALS**

Weight: 22g (thin slice)

15g CARBS   **72 CALS**

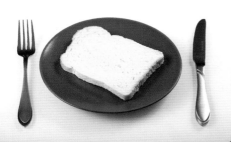

Weight: 33g (medium slice)

20g CARBS   **94 CALS**

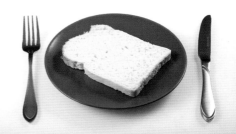

Weight: 43g (thick slice)

30g CARBS   **140 CALS**

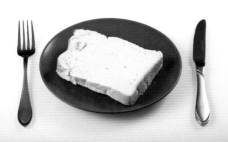

Weight: 64g (extra thick slice)

39g CARBS   **186 CALS**

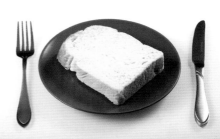

Weight: 85g

Sliced Bread (wholemeal)

5g CARBS | **24 CALS**

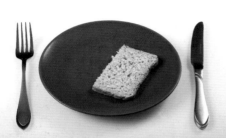

Weight: 11g (thin slice)

10g CARBS | **50 CALS**

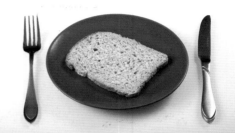

Weight: 23g (thin slice)

15g CARBS | **78 CALS**

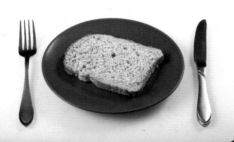

Weight: 36g (medium slice)

21g CARBS | **106 CALS**

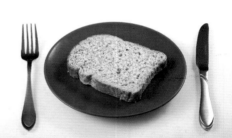

Weight: 49g (thick slice)

30g CARBS | **154 CALS**

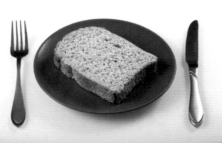

Weight: 71g (extra thick slice)

40g CARBS | **206 CALS**

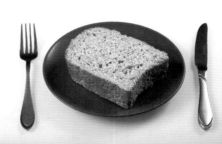

Weight: 95g

Bap (white)

25g CARBS | **122 CALS**

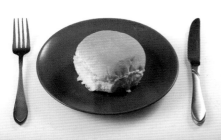

Weight: 48g

60g CARBS | **295 CALS**

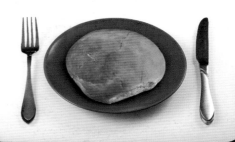

Weight: 116g

Bap (wholemeal)

24g CARBS | **124 CALS**

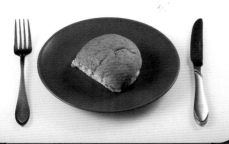

Weight: 51g

53g CARBS | **278 CALS**

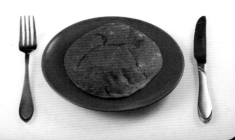

Weight: 114g

Crusty Roll (white)

24g CARBS | **113 CALS**

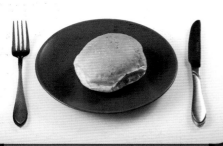

Weight: 43g

47g CARBS | **225 CALS**

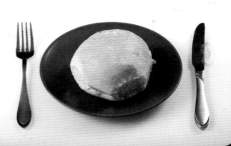

Weight: 86g

Bagel

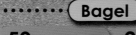

50g CARBS   **235** CALS

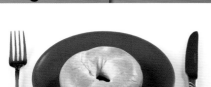

Weight: 86g

Burger Bun

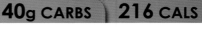

40g CARBS   **216** CALS

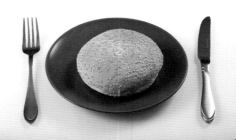

Weight: 82g

Finger Roll

21g CARBS   **104** CALS

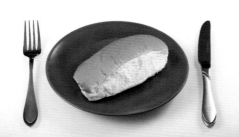

Weight: 41g

Poppy Seeded Roll

26g CARBS   **152** CALS

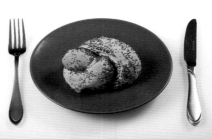

Weight: 54g

Pitta Bread

38g CARBS   **176** CALS

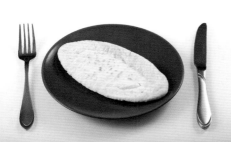

Weight: 69g

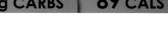

19g CARBS   **89** CALS

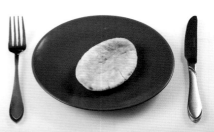

Weight: 35g (mini)

Ciabatta

50g CARBS | **263** CALS

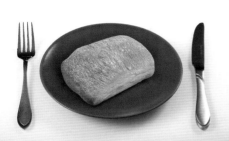

Weight: 97g

Panini

45g CARBS | **278** CALS

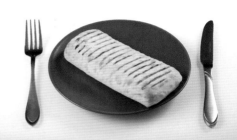

Weight: 100g

French Stick

21g CARBS | **97** CALS

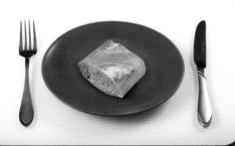

Weight: 37g (slice)

66g CARBS | **310** CALS

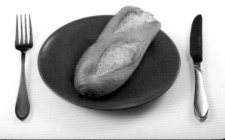

Weight: 118g (small)

Garlic Bread

10g CARBS | **80** CALS

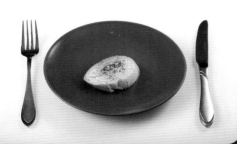

Weight: 22g

30g CARBS | **241** CALS

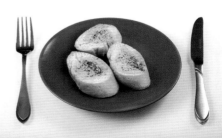

Weight: 66g

Crumpet

20g CARBS   **93 CALS**

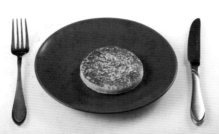

Weight: 45g

26g CARBS   **118 CALS**

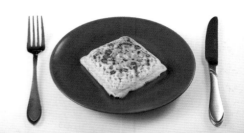

Weight: 57g (square)

English Muffin

35g CARBS   **177 CALS**

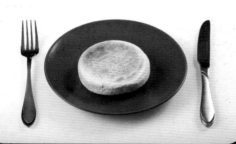

Weight: 68g

Tea Cake

50g CARBS   **280 CALS**

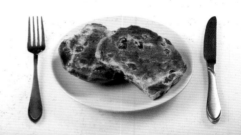

Weight: 85g

Tortilla

35g CARBS   **152 CALS**

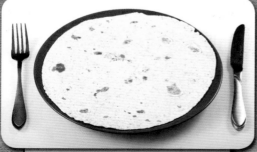

Weight: 58g

Turkish Flatbread

27g CARBS   **153 CALS**

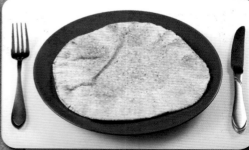

Weight: 60g

Naan Bread

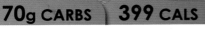

70g CARBS | **399 CALS**

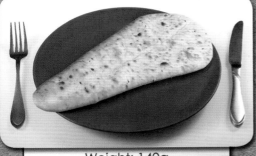

Weight: 140g

30g CARBS | **171 CALS**

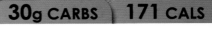

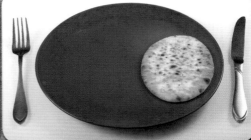

Weight: 60g (mini)

Chapati (without fat)

20g CARBS | **91 CALS**

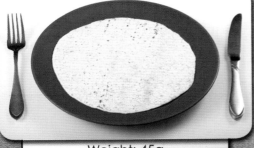

Weight: 45g

Paratha

40g CARBS | **297 CALS**

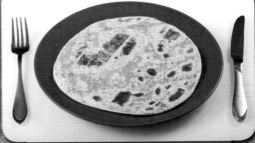

Weight: 92g

Poppadom

4g CARBS | **65 CALS**

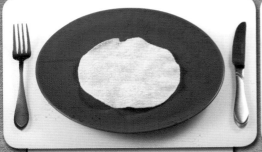

Weight: 13g (small)

7g CARBS | **125 CALS**

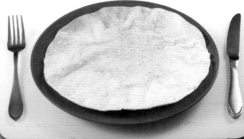

Weight: 25g (large)

Brioche

10g CARBS   **64 CALS**   **25g CARBS**   **159 CALS**

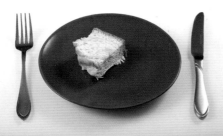

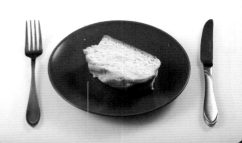

Weight: 18g

Weight: 45g

Croissant

11g CARBS   **97 CALS**   **22g CARBS**   **190 CALS**

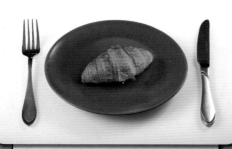

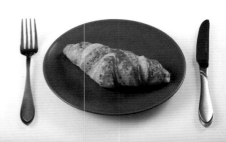

Weight: 26g

Weight: 51g

Pain au Chocolat

14g CARBS   **142 CALS**   **27g CARBS**   **267 CALS**

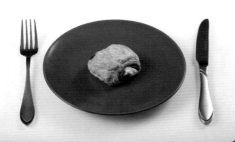

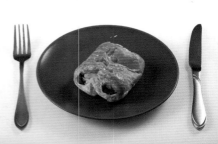

Weight: 32g

Weight: 64g

Toast with Chocolate Spread & Margarine

7g CARBS   57 CALS

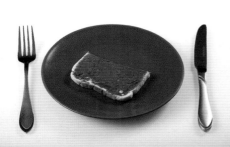

	CARBS	CALS
2x	14g	114
3x	21g	171
4x	28g	228

8g toast, 2g choc, 2g marg

13g CARBS   112 CALS

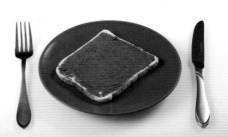

	CARBS	CALS
2x	26g	224
3x	39g	336
4x	52g	448

16g toast, 5g choc, 5g marg

18g CARBS   136 CALS

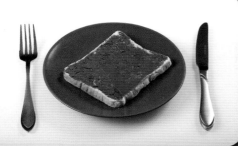

	CARBS	CALS
2x	36g	272
3x	54g	408
4x	72g	544

26g toast, 5g choc, 5g marg

23g CARBS   158 CALS

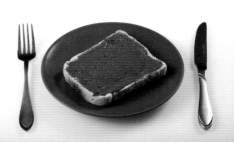

	CARBS	CALS
2x	46g	316
3x	69g	474
4x	92g	632

36g toast, 5g choc, 5g marg

Toast with Honey & Margarine

7g CARBS   **50 CALS**

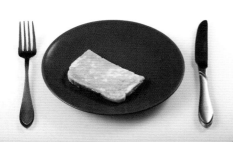

	CARBS	CALS
2x	14g	100
3x	21g	150
4x	28g	200

8g toast, 2g honey, 2g marg

14g CARBS   **99 CALS**

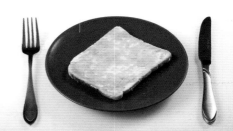

	CARBS	CALS
2x	28g	198
3x	42g	297
4x	56g	396

16g toast, 5g honey, 5g marg

19g CARBS   **123 CALS**

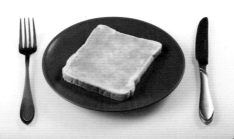

	CARBS	CALS
2x	38g	246
3x	57g	369
4x	76g	492

26g toast, 5g honey, 5g marg

24g CARBS   **145 CALS**

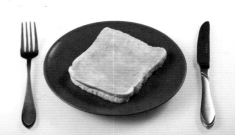

	CARBS	CALS
2x	48g	290
3x	72g	435
4x	96g	580

36g toast, 5g honey, 5g marg

Toast with Jam & Margarine

7g CARBS   50 CALS

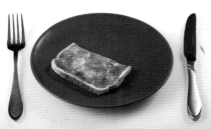

	CARBS	CALS
2x	14g	100
3x	21g	150
4x	28g	200

8g toast, 2g jam, 2g marg

13g CARBS   98 CALS

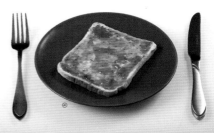

	CARBS	CALS
2x	26g	196
3x	39g	294
4x	52g	392

16g toast, 5g jam, 5g marg

18g CARBS   122 CALS

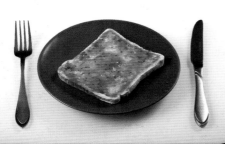

	CARBS	CALS
2x	36g	244
3x	54g	366
4x	72g	488

26g toast, 5g jam, 5g marg

23g CARBS   144 CALS

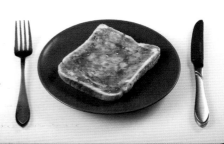

	CARBS	CALS
2x	46g	288
3x	69g	432
4x	92g	576

36g toast, 5g jam, 5g marg

Toast with Lemon Curd & Margarine

7g CARBS   50 CALS

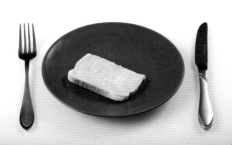

	CARBS	CALS
2x	14g	100
3x	21g	150
4x	28g	200

8g toast, 2g curd, 2g marg

13g CARBS   99 CALS

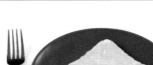
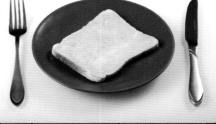

	CARBS	CALS
2x	26g	198
3x	39g	297
4x	52g	396

16g toast, 5g curd, 5g marg

18g CARBS   123 CALS

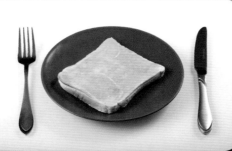

	CARBS	CALS
2x	36g	246
3x	54g	369
4x	72g	492

26g toast, 5g curd, 5g marg

23g CARBS   145 CALS

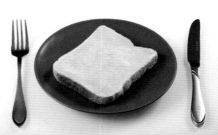

	CARBS	CALS
2x	46g	290
3x	69g	435
4x	92g	580

36g toast, 5g curd, 5g marg

Toast with Marmalade & Margarine

7g CARBS   **50 CALS**

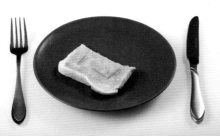

	CARBS	CALS
2x	14g	100
3x	21g	150
4x	28g	200

8g toast, 2g marm, 2g marg

13g CARBS   **98 CALS**

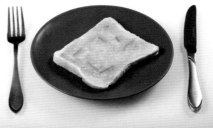

	CARBS	CALS
2x	26g	196
3x	39g	294
4x	52g	392

16g toast, 5g marm, 5g marg

18g CARBS   **122 CALS**

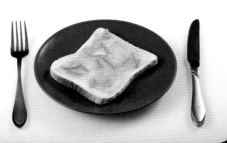

	CARBS	CALS
2x	36g	244
3x	54g	366
4x	72g	488

26g toast, 5g marm, 5g marg

23g CARBS   **144 CALS**

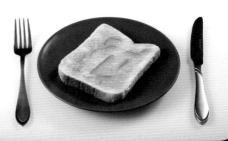
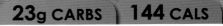

	CARBS	CALS
2x	46g	288
3x	69g	432
4x	92g	576

36g toast, 5g marm, 5g marg

Toast with Peanut Butter & Margarine

5g CARBS · 58 CALS

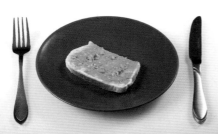

	CARBS	CALS
2x	10g	116
3x	15g	174
4x	20g	232

8g toast, 2g peanut, 2g marg

11g CARBS · 115 CALS

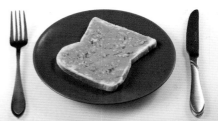

	CARBS	CALS
2x	22g	230
3x	33g	345
4x	44g	460

16g toast, 5g peanut, 5g marg

16g CARBS · 139 CALS

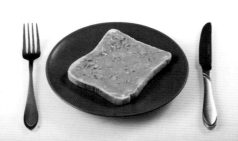

	CARBS	CALS
2x	32g	278
3x	48g	417
4x	64g	556

26g toast, 5g peanut, 5g marg

21g CARBS · 161 CALS

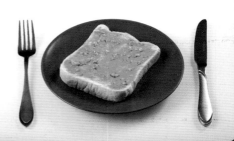

	CARBS	CALS
2x	42g	322
3x	63g	483
4x	84g	644

36g toast, 5g peanut, 5g marg

Bran Flakes

11g CARBS · **50 CALS**

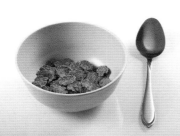

Weight: 15g

21g CARBS · **99 CALS**

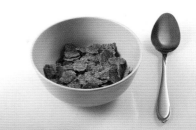

Weight: 30g

32g CARBS · **149 CALS**

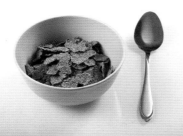

Weight: 45g

43g CARBS · **198 CALS**

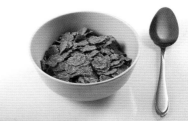

Weight: 60g

53g CARBS · **248 CALS**

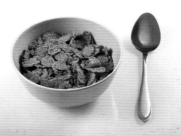

Weight: 75g

65g CARBS · **300 CALS**

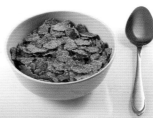

Weight: 91g

Chocolate Snaps

10g CARBS   **42 CALS**

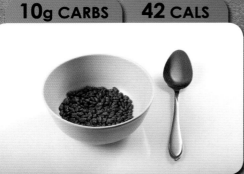

Weight: 11g

19g CARBS   **80 CALS**

Weight: 21g

29g CARBS   **123 CALS**

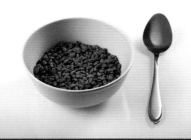

Weight: 32g

38g CARBS   **161 CALS**

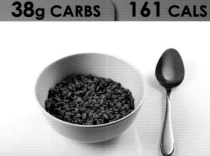

Weight: 42g

48g CARBS   **203 CALS**

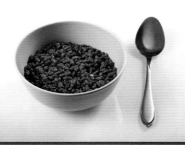

Weight: 53g

59g CARBS   **245 CALS**

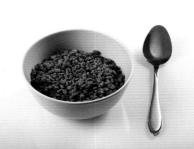

Weight: 64g

Corn Flakes

11g CARBS   **45 CALS**

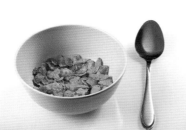

Weight: 12g

21g CARBS   **86 CALS**

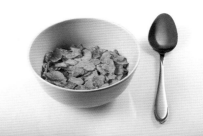

Weight: 23g

31g CARBS   **132 CALS**

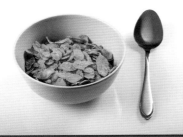

Weight: 35g

42g CARBS   **177 CALS**

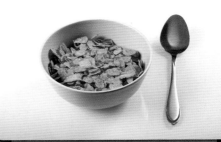

Weight: 47g

52g CARBS   **218 CALS**

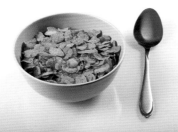

Weight: 58g

63g CARBS   **263 CALS**

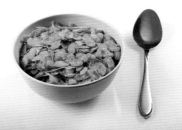

Weight: 70g

Fruit & Fibre

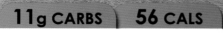

11g CARBS | **56 CALS**

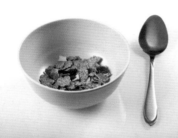

Weight: 15g

21g CARBS | **107 CALS**

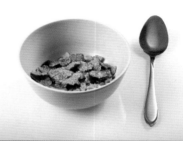

Weight: 29g

32g CARBS | **163 CALS**

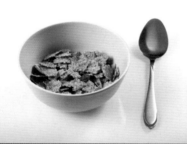

Weight: 44g

43g CARBS | **218 CALS**

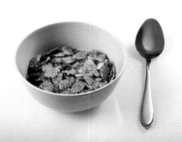

Weight: 59g

53g CARBS | **270 CALS**

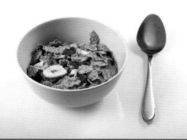

Weight: 73g

64g CARBS | **326 CALS**

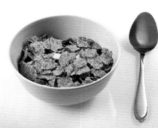

Weight: 88g

Honey Puffed Wheat

11g CARBS | **46 CALS**

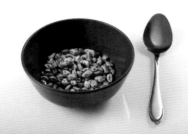

Weight: 12g

21g CARBS | **88 CALS**

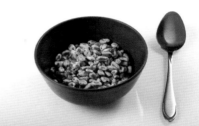

Weight: 23g

32g CARBS | **133 CALS**

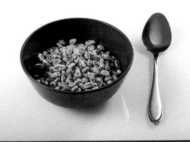

Weight: 35g

44g CARBS | **179 CALS**

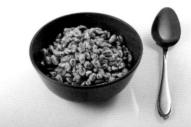

Weight: 47g

54g CARBS | **221 CALS**

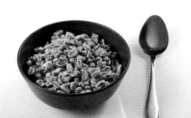

Weight: 58g

65g CARBS | **267 CALS**

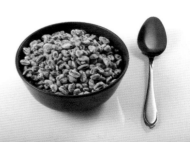

Weight: 70g

Malted Wheats

11g CARBS **48 CALS**

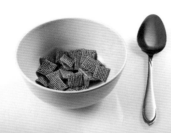

Weight: 14g

22g CARBS **97 CALS**

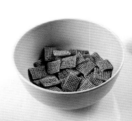

Weight: 28g

32g CARBS **145 CALS**

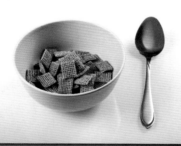

Weight: 42g

43g CARBS **194 CALS**

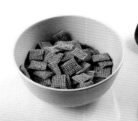

Weight: 56g

54g CARBS **242 CALS**

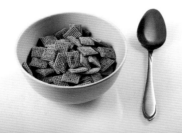

Weight: 70g

65g CARBS **291 CALS**

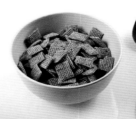

Weight: 84g

Muesli

22g CARBS   **109** CALS

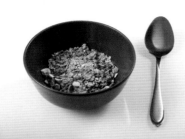

Weight: 30g

43g CARBS   **218** CALS

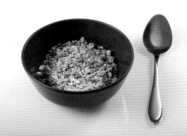

Weight: 60g

65g CARBS   **327** CALS

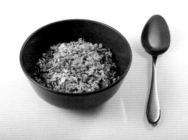

Weight: 90g

86g CARBS   **432** CALS

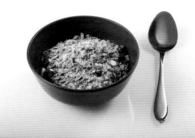

Weight: 119g

108g CARBS   **541** CALS

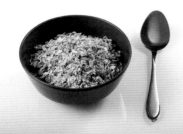

Weight: 149g

129g CARBS   **650** CALS

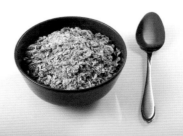

Weight: 179g

Multigrain Hoops

10g CARBS   **48 CALS**

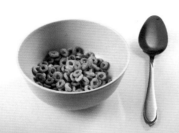

Weight: 13g

16g CARBS   **74 CALS**

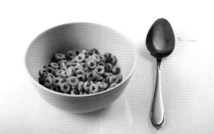

Weight: 20g

22g CARBS   **99 CALS**

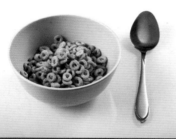

Weight: 27g

27g CARBS   **121 CALS**

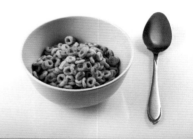

Weight: 33g

32g CARBS   **147 CALS**

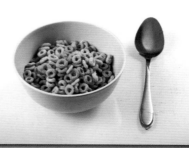

Weight: 40g

38g CARBS   **173 CALS**

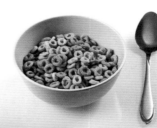

Weight: 47g

Porridge (made with whole milk)

9g CARBS | **85 CALS**

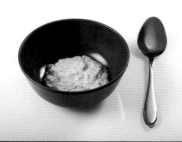

Weight: 75g

18g CARBS | **164 CALS**

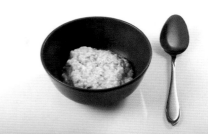

Weight: 145g

28g CARBS | **249 CALS**

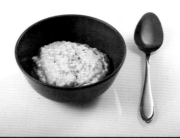

Weight: 220g

37g CARBS | **328 CALS**

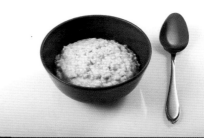

Weight: 290g

46g CARBS | **412 CALS**

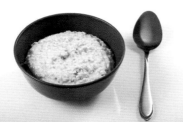

Weight: 365g

55g CARBS | **492 CALS**

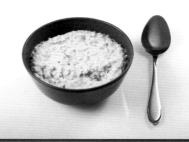

Weight: 435g

Raisin Bites

17g CARBS | **74 CALS**

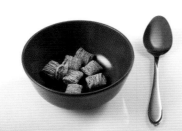

Weight: 22g

33g CARBS | **148 CALS**

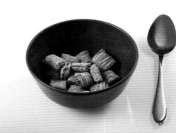

Weight: 44g

49g CARBS | **219 CALS**

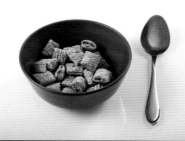

Weight: 65g

66g CARBS | **293 CALS**

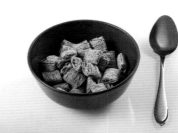

Weight: 87g

81g CARBS | **364 CALS**

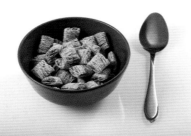

Weight: 108g

98g CARBS | **438 CALS**

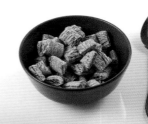

Weight: 130g

Rice Snaps

10g CARBS | **42** CALS

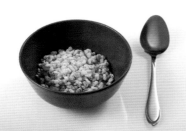

Weight: 11g

21g CARBS | **88** CALS

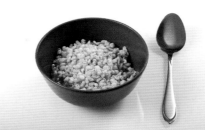

Weight: 23g

32g CARBS | **130** CALS

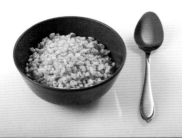

Weight: 34g

43g CARBS | **176** CALS

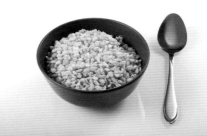

Weight: 46g

53g CARBS | **218** CALS

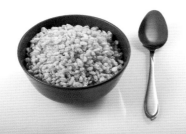

Weight: 57g

64g CARBS | **264** CALS

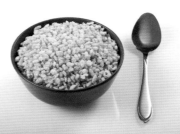

Weight: 69g

Special Flakes with Berries

10g CARBS | **48 CALS**

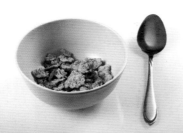

Weight: 13g

20g CARBS | **97 CALS**

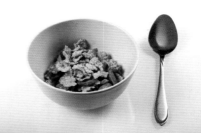

Weight: 26g

31g CARBS | **149 CALS**

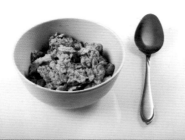

Weight: 40g

41g CARBS | **198 CALS**

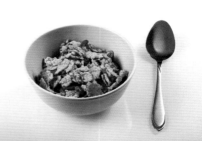

Weight: 53g

51g CARBS | **246 CALS**

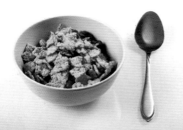

Weight: 66g

62g CARBS | **298 CALS**

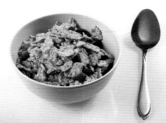

Weight: 80g

Wheat Biscuit

14g CARBS | **67** CALS

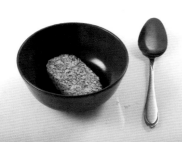

	CARBS	CALS
2x	28g	134
3x	42g	201
4x	56g	268
Weight: 19g		

Wheat Pillow

16g CARBS | **73** CALS

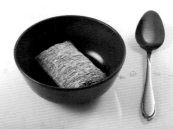

	CARBS	CALS
2x	32g	146
3x	48g	219
4x	64g	292
Weight: 22g		

Oat Biscuit

13g CARBS | **75** CALS

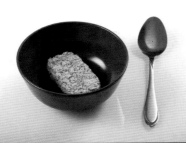

	CARBS	CALS
2x	26g	150
3x	39g	225
4x	52g	300
Weight: 20g		

Milk (semi-skimmed)

5g CARBS | **46** CALS

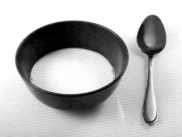

	CARBS	CALS
2x	10g	92
3x	15g	138
4x	20g	184
Weight: 100g		

Eggy Bread

5g CARBS **97 CALS**

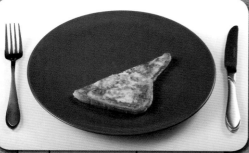

	CARBS	CALS
2x	10g	194
3x	15g	291
4x	20g	388
Weight: 25g (thin slice)		

10g CARBS **193 CALS**

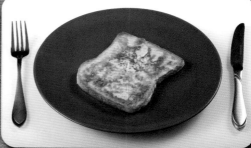

	CARBS	CALS
2x	20g	386
3x	30g	579
4x	40g	772
Weight: 50g (thin slice)		

Fried Bread

5g CARBS **80 CALS**

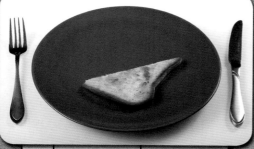

	CARBS	CALS
2x	10g	160
3x	15g	240
4x	20g	320
Weight: 15g (thin slice)		

10g CARBS **160 CALS**

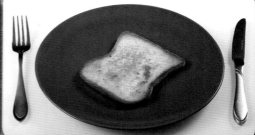

	CARBS	CALS
2x	20g	320
3x	30g	480
4x	40g	640
Weight: 30g (thin slice)		

Breakfast Tart

36g CARBS   **211 CALS**

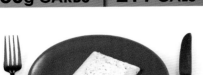

	CARBS	CALS
2x	72g	422
3x	108g	633
4x	144g	844
Weight: 52g		

Scotch Pancake

12g CARBS   **88 CALS**

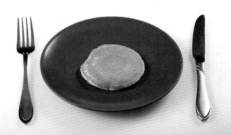

	CARBS	CALS
2x	24g	176
3x	36g	264
4x	48g	352
Weight: 31g		

Waffle (sweet)

15g CARBS   **129 CALS**

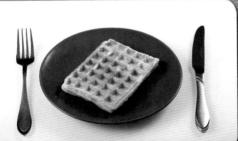

	CARBS	CALS
2x	30g	258
3x	45g	387
4x	60g	516
Weight: 38g		

24g CARBS   **201 CALS**

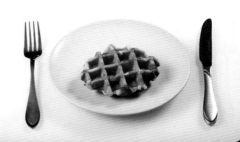

	CARBS	CALS
2x	48g	402
3x	72g	603
4x	96g	804
Weight: 59g		

Pancake (plain)

5g CARBS   56 CALS

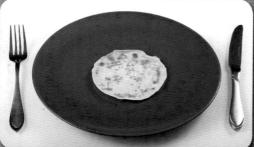

	CARBS	CALS
2x	10g	112
3x	15g	168
4x	20g	224
Weight: 22g		

10g CARBS   110 CALS

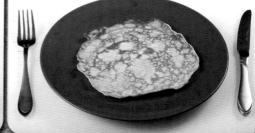

	CARBS	CALS
2x	20g	220
3x	30g	330
4x	40g	440
Weight: 43g		

15g CARBS   158 CALS

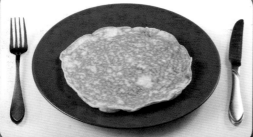

	CARBS	CALS
2x	30g	316
3x	45g	474
4x	60g	632
Weight: 62g		

20g CARBS   217 CALS

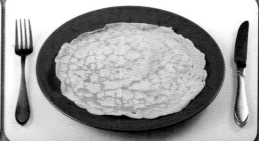

	CARBS	CALS
2x	40g	434
3x	60g	651
4x	80g	868
Weight: 85g		

Pancake with Chocolate Spread

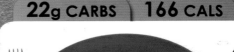

14g CARBS | 106 CALS

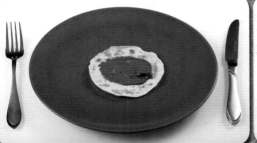

	CARBS	CALS
2x	28g	212
3x	42g	318
4x	56g	424

22g pancake, 8g chocolate

22g CARBS | 166 CALS

	CARBS	CALS
2x	44g	332
3x	66g	498
4x	88g	664

43g pancake, 8g chocolate

34g CARBS | 264 CALS

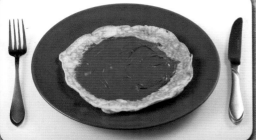

	CARBS	CALS
2x	68g	528
3x	102g	792
4x	136g	1056

62g pancake, 16g chocolate

44g CARBS | 329 CALS

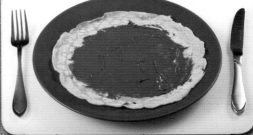

	CARBS	CALS
2x	88g	658
3x	132g	987
4x	176g	1316

85g pancake, 16g chocolate

Pancake with Maple Syrup

14g CARBS   **83 CALS**

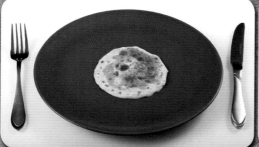

	CARBS	CALS
2x	28g	166
3x	42g	249
4x	56g	332
22g pancake, 8g syrup		

22g CARBS   **143 CALS**

	CARBS	CALS
2x	44g	286
3x	66g	429
4x	88g	572
43g pancake, 8g syrup		

35g CARBS   **218 CALS**

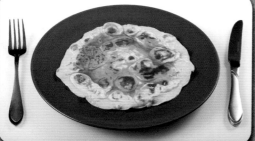

	CARBS	CALS
2x	70g	436
3x	105g	654
4x	140g	872
62 pancake, 16g syrup		

45g CARBS   **283 CALS**

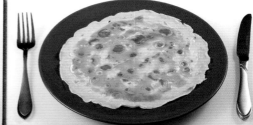

	CARBS	CALS
2x	90g	566
3x	135g	849
4x	180g	1132
85g pancake, 16g syrup		

Pancake with Sugar & Lemon

14g CARBS · 82 CALS

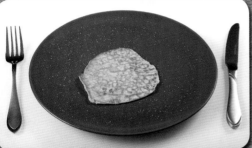

	CARBS	CALS
2x	28g	164
3x	42g	246
4x	56g	328
22g pancake, 5g sugar		

22g CARBS · 142 CALS

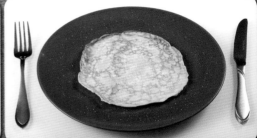

	CARBS	CALS
2x	44g	284
3x	66g	426
4x	88g	568
43g pancake, 5g sugar		

35g CARBS · 215 CALS

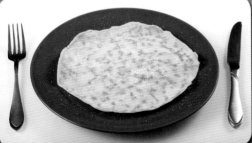

	CARBS	CALS
2x	70g	430
3x	105g	645
4x	140g	860
62g pancake, 10g sugar		

45g CARBS · 280 CALS

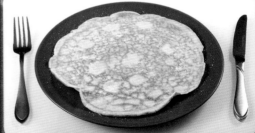

	CARBS	CALS
2x	90g	560
3x	135g	840
4x	180g	1120
85g pancake, 10g sugar		

Greek Yoghurt

4g CARBS | **113 CALS**

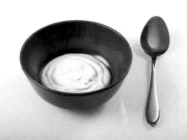

Weight: 85g

8g CARBS | **226 CALS**

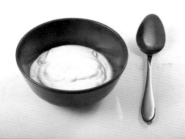

Weight: 170g

12g CARBS | **346 CALS**

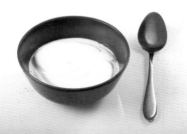

Weight: 260g

Natural Yoghurt

5g CARBS | **55 CALS**

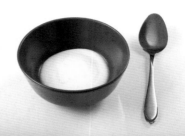

Weight: 70g

15g CARBS | **150 CALS**

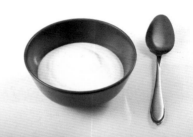

Weight: 190g

25g CARBS | **253 CALS**

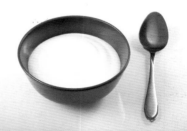

Weight: 320g

Baklava

9g CARBS | 79 CALS

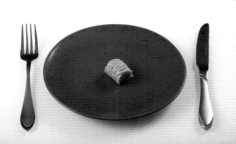

	CARBS	CALS
2x	18g	158
3x	27g	237
4x	36g	316
Weight: 20g		

13g CARBS | 110 CALS

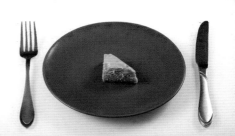

	CARBS	CALS
2x	26g	220
3x	39g	330
4x	52g	440
Weight: 28g		

6g CARBS | 55 CALS

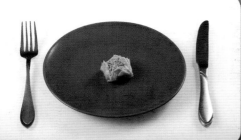

	CARBS	CALS
2x	12g	110
3x	18g	165
4x	24g	220
Weight: 14g		

12g CARBS | 102 CALS

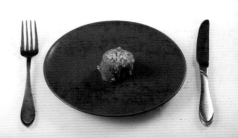

	CARBS	CALS
2x	24g	204
3x	36g	306
4x	48g	408
Weight: 26g		

Bakewell Tart

15g CARBS   **155 CALS**

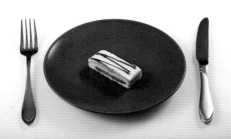

Weight: 34g

20g CARBS   **205 CALS**

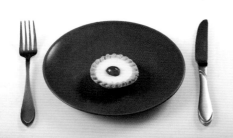

Weight: 45g

40g CARBS   **424 CALS**

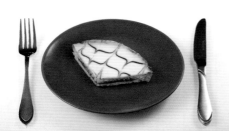

Weight: 93g

Carrot Cake

20g CARBS   **190 CALS**

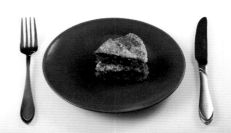

Weight: 53g

40g CARBS   **384 CALS**

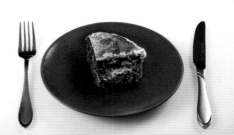

Weight: 107g

60g CARBS   **578 CALS**

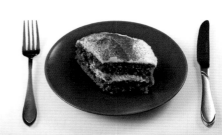

Weight: 161g

Chocolate Cake

20g CARBS   **186 CALS**

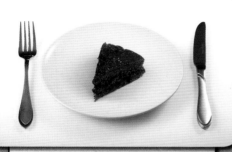

Weight: 40g

35g CARBS   **325 CALS**

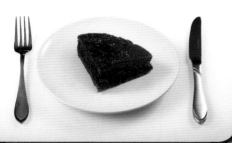

Weight: 70g

70g CARBS   **640 CALS**

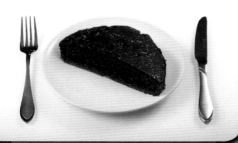

Weight: 138g

Fruit Cake

16g CARBS   **89 CALS**

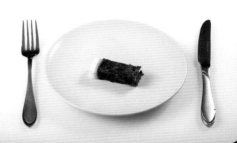

Weight: 26g

36g CARBS   **206 CALS**

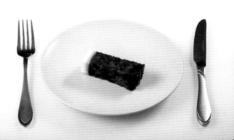

Weight: 60g

72g CARBS   **415 CALS**

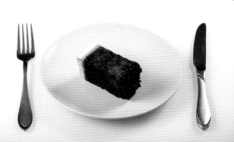

Weight: 121g

Ginger Cake

15g CARBS   **86** CALS

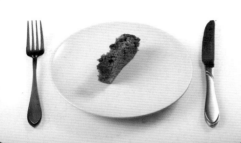

Weight: 24g

25g CARBS   **144** CALS

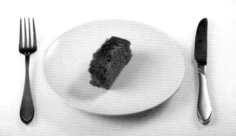

Weight: 40g

35g CARBS   **202** CALS

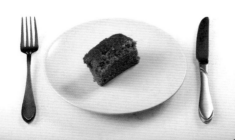

Weight: 56g

Malt Loaf

19g CARBS   **89** CALS

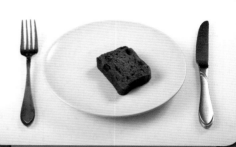

Weight: 30g

40g CARBS   **180** CALS

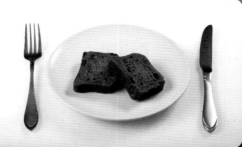

Weight: 61g

59g CARBS   **268** CALS

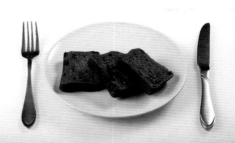

Weight: 91g

Swiss Roll

17g CARBS　**134 CALS**

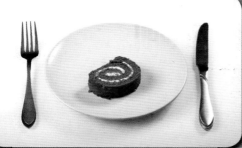

Weight: 35g

33g CARBS　**264 CALS**

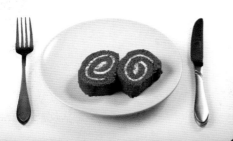

Weight: 69g

49g CARBS　**394 CALS**

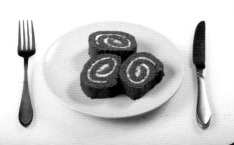

Weight: 103g

Victoria Sponge

19g CARBS　**123 CALS**

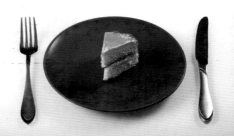

Weight: 44g

34g CARBS　**216 CALS**

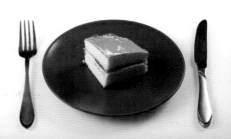

Weight: 77g

68g CARBS　**434 CALS**

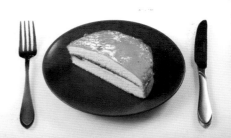

Weight: 155g

Apple Danish

45g CARBS | **298** CALS

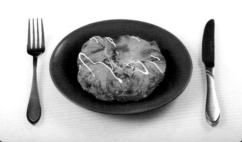

Weight: 87g

Choc Chip Twist

40g CARBS | **357** CALS

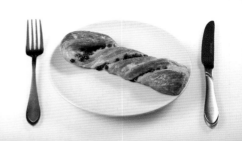

Weight: 85g

Cinnamon Swirl

41g CARBS | **270** CALS

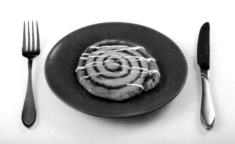

Weight: 79g

Fruit Trellis

28g CARBS | **206** CALS

Weight: 58g

Pain au Raisin

44g CARBS | **364** CALS

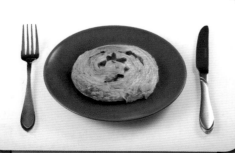

Weight: 95g

Pecan Plait

36g CARBS | **347** CALS

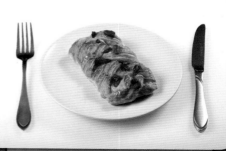

Weight: 81g

Chocolate Éclair

21g CARBS | **217 CALS**

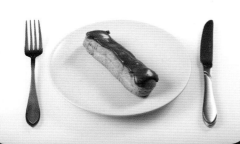

Weight: 56g

Corn Flake Cake

35g CARBS | **248 CALS**

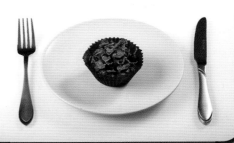

Weight: 54g

Cup Cake

34g CARBS | **272 CALS**

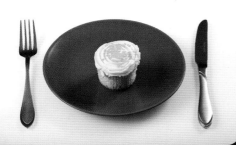

Weight: 56g

Custard Slice

40g CARBS | **286 CALS**

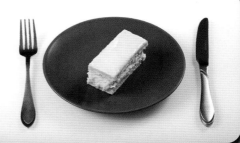

Weight: 106g

Custard Tart

26g CARBS | **263 CALS**

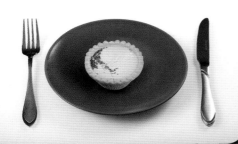

Weight: 92g

Mini Battenburg

16g CARBS | **112 CALS**

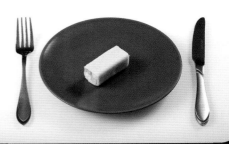

Weight: 30g

20cm Side Plate

Choc Ring Doughnut

25g CARBS | **201 CALS**

Weight: 49g

Glazed Ring Doughnut

25g CARBS | **176 CALS**

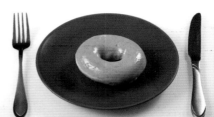

Weight: 46g

Jam Doughnut

35g CARBS | **239 CALS**

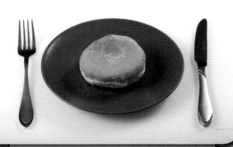

Weight: 71g

Mini Doughnut

6g CARBS | **45 CALS**

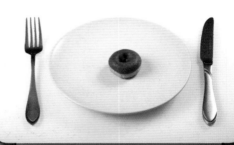

Weight: 11g

Sprinkle Ring Doughnut

32g CARBS | **240 CALS**

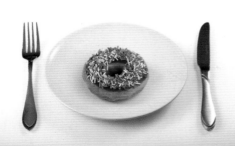

Weight: 58g

Sugar Ring Doughnut

31g CARBS | **266 CALS**

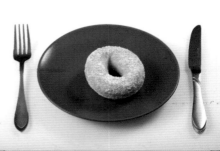

Weight: 66g

Fresh Cream Doughnut

25g CARBS | **221** CALS

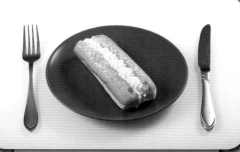

Weight: 69g

Yum Yum

32g CARBS | **276** CALS

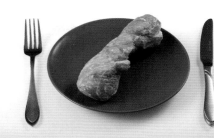

Weight: 70g

Blueberry Muffin

12g CARBS | **86** CALS

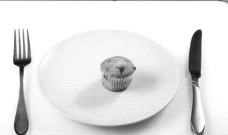

Weight: 25g

48g CARBS | **353** CALS

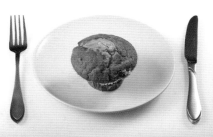

Weight: 102g

Chocolate Muffin

15g CARBS | **108** CALS

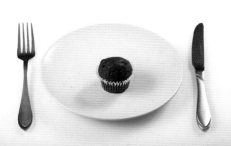

Weight: 28g

55g CARBS | **404** CALS

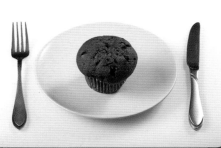

Weight: 105g

Flapjack

31g CARBS   **247** CALS   **51**g CARBS   **404** CALS

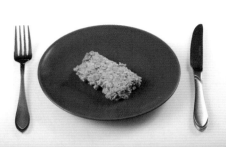

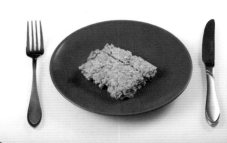

Weight: 50g   Weight: 82g

Meringue Nest

5g CARBS   **19** CALS   **15**g CARBS   **61** CALS

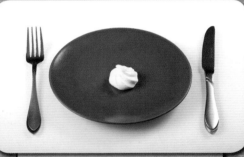

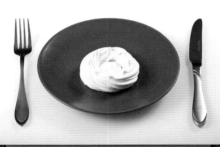

Weight: 5g   Weight: 16g

Mince Pie

25g CARBS   **183** CALS   **36**g CARBS   **261** CALS

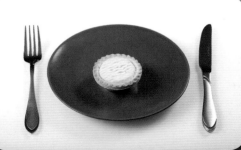

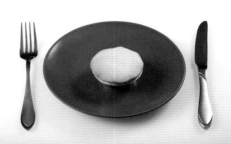

Weight: 42g   Weight: 60g

Belgian Bun

69g CARBS | **411** CALS

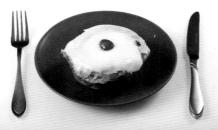

Weight: 116g

Cheese Scone

30g CARBS | **251** CALS

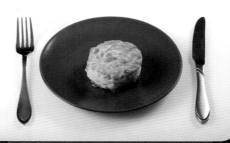

Weight: 68g

Fruit Scone

21g CARBS | **120** CALS

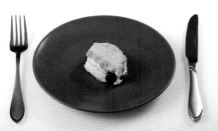

Weight: 38g

37g CARBS | **208** CALS

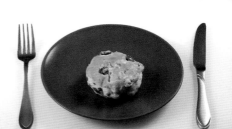

Weight: 66g

Hot Cross Bun

30g CARBS | **159** CALS

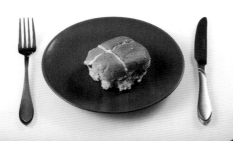

Weight: 51g

Iced Bun

20g CARBS | **113** CALS

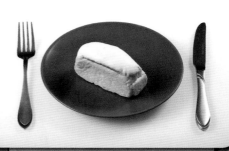

Weight: 37g

Apple Pie

18g CARBS   **134** CALS

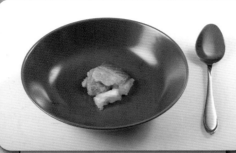

Weight: 50g

36g CARBS   **267** CALS

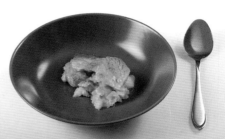

Weight: 100g

54g CARBS   **403** CALS

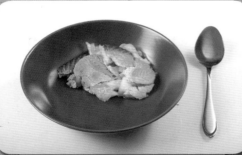

Weight: 151g

72g CARBS   **537** CALS

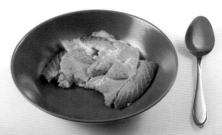

Weight: 201g

90g CARBS   **673** CALS

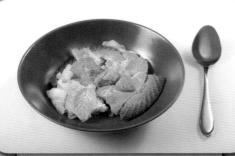

Weight: 252g

108g CARBS   **806** CALS

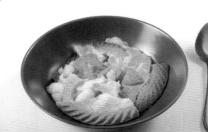

Weight: 302g

Apple & Rhubarb Crumble

22g CARBS   **131** CALS

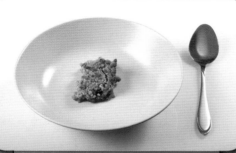

Weight: 60g

42g CARBS   **256** CALS

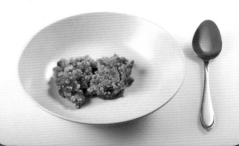

Weight: 117g

63g CARBS   **383** CALS

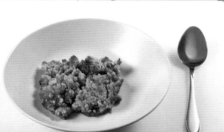

Weight: 175g

85g CARBS   **515** CALS

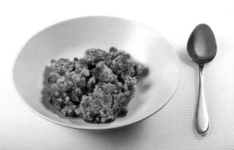

Weight: 235g

106g CARBS   **646** CALS

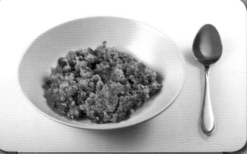

Weight: 295g

127g CARBS   **771** CALS

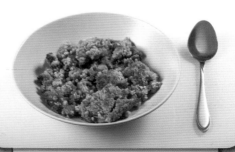

Weight: 352g

Apple Strudel

14g CARBS | **110 CALS**

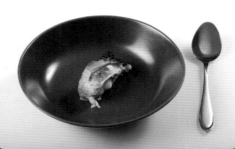

Weight: 45g

28g CARBS | **221 CALS**

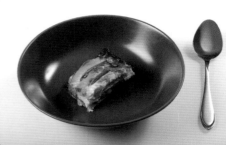

Weight: 90g

42g CARBS | **331 CALS**

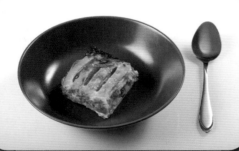

Weight: 135g

56g CARBS | **446 CALS**

Weight: 182g

70g CARBS | **559 CALS**

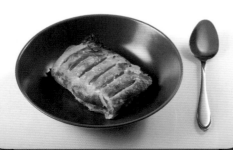

Weight: 228g

84g CARBS | **666 CALS**

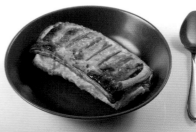

Weight: 272g

Banoffee Pie

14g CARBS | **137 CALS**

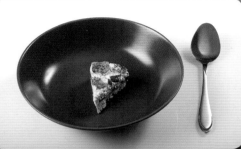

Weight: 43g

29g CARBS | **284 CALS**

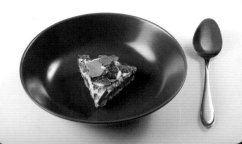

Weight: 89g

44g CARBS | **424 CALS**

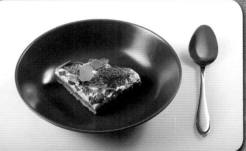

Weight: 133g

58g CARBS | **561 CALS**

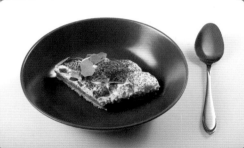

Weight: 176g

72g CARBS | **702 CALS**

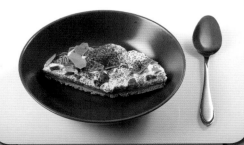

Weight: 220g

87g CARBS | **845 CALS**

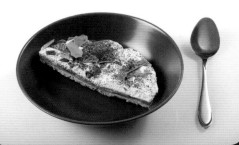

Weight: 265g

Black Forest Gateau

13g CARBS   **103 CALS**

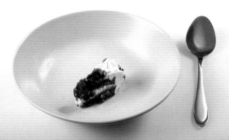

Weight: 35g

25g CARBS   **201 CALS**

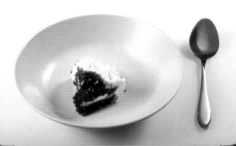

Weight: 68g

37g CARBS   **295 CALS**

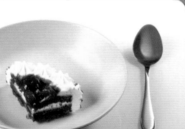

Weight: 100g

50g CARBS   **398 CALS**

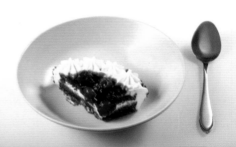

Weight: 135g

62g CARBS   **496 CALS**

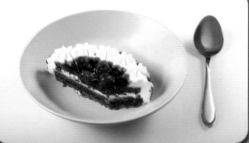

Weight: 168g

74g CARBS   **590 CALS**

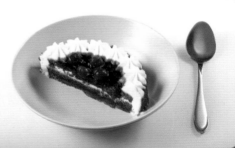

Weight: 200g

Bread & Butter Pudding

10g CARBS | **98 CALS**

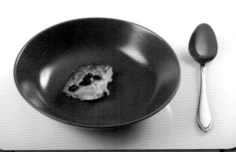

Weight: 40g

19g CARBS | **199 CALS**

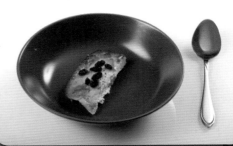

Weight: 81g

29g CARBS | **300 CALS**

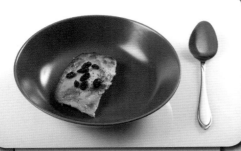

Weight: 122g

39g CARBS | **403 CALS**

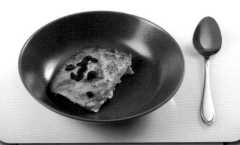

Weight: 164g

49g CARBS | **504 CALS**

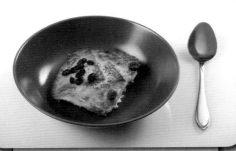

Weight: 205g

59g CARBS | **605 CALS**

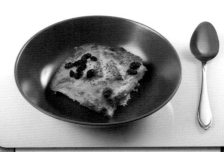

Weight: 246g

Brownie

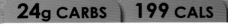

24g CARBS   **199 CALS**

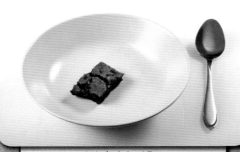

Weight: 45g

43g CARBS   **362 CALS**

Weight: 82g

67g CARBS   **561 CALS**

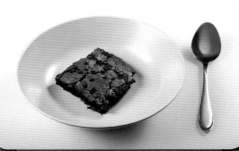

Weight: 127g

87g CARBS   **725 CALS**

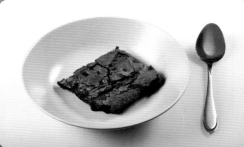

Weight: 164g

111g CARBS   **924 CALS**

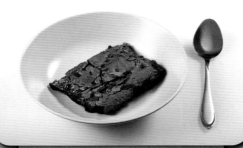

Weight: 209g

130g CARBS   **1087 CALS**

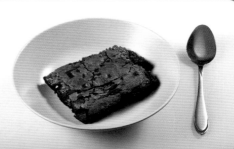

Weight: 246g

Cheesecake

18g CARBS   **147 CALS**

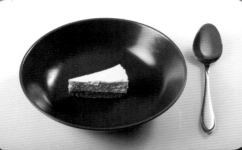

Weight: 50g

35g CARBS   **294 CALS**

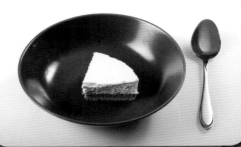

Weight: 100g

53g CARBS   **441 CALS**

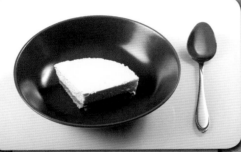

Weight: 150g

70g CARBS   **588 CALS**

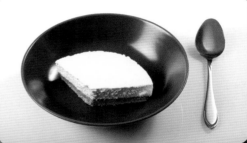

Weight: 200g

88g CARBS   **735 CALS**

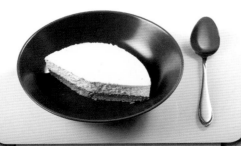

Weight: 250g

106g CARBS   **882 CALS**

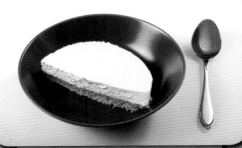

Weight: 300g

Chocolate Torte

11g CARBS   **140 CALS**

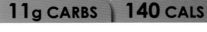

Weight: 33g

21g CARBS   **279 CALS**

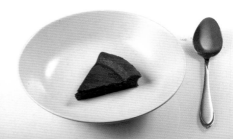

Weight: 66g

32g CARBS   **423 CALS**

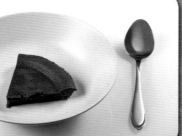

Weight: 100g

43g CARBS   **563 CALS**

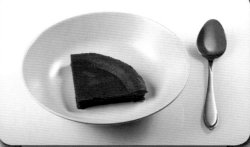

Weight: 133g

53g CARBS   **702 CALS**

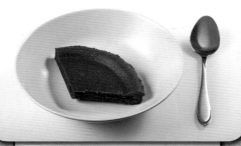

Weight: 166g

64g CARBS   **846 CALS**

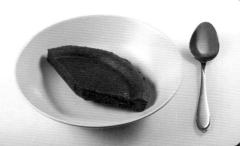

Weight: 200g

Christmas Pudding

20g CARBS   **115 CALS**

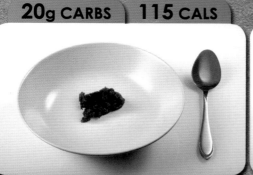

Weight: 35g

40g CARBS   **234 CALS**

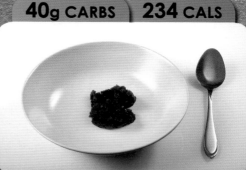

Weight: 71g

60g CARBS   **349 CALS**

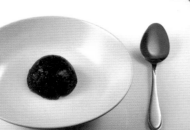

Weight: 106g (individual)

80g CARBS   **467 CALS**

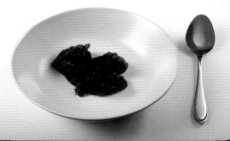

Weight: 142g

100g CARBS   **582 CALS**

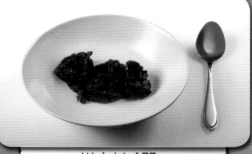

Weight: 177g

120g CARBS   **704 CALS**

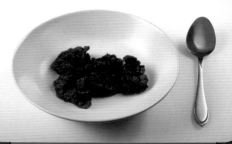

Weight: 214g

Custard (made with whole milk)

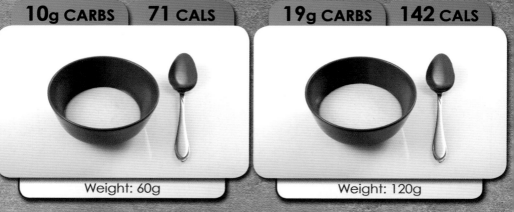

| 10g CARBS | 71 CALS | 19g CARBS | 142 CALS |

Weight: 60g

Weight: 120g

| 29g CARBS | 212 CALS | 39g CARBS | 283 CALS |

Weight: 180g

Weight: 240g

| 49g CARBS | 354 CALS | 58g CARBS | 425 CALS |

Weight: 300g

Weight: 360g

Ice Cream (vanilla)

8g CARBS | **71 CALS**

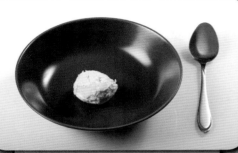

Weight: 40g

16g CARBS | **142 CALS**

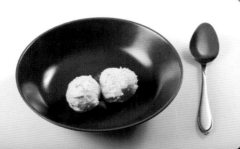

Weight: 80g

24g CARBS | **214 CALS**

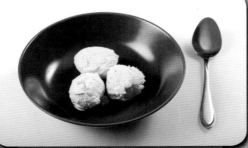

Weight: 121g

Lemon Sorbet

11g CARBS | **44 CALS**

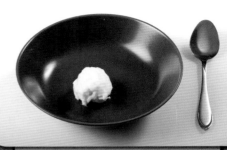

Weight: 45g

22g CARBS | **85 CALS**

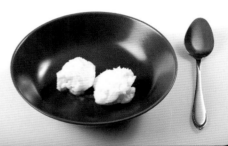

Weight: 88g

33g CARBS | **128 CALS**

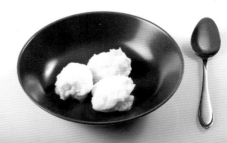

Weight: 132g

Choc Ice

12g CARBS | **153 CALS**

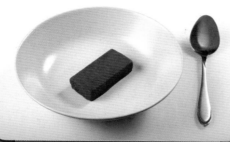

Weight: 52g

Crème Brûlée

15g CARBS | **343 CALS**

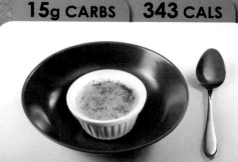

Weight: 104g

Chocolate & Nut Cone

21g CARBS | **207 CALS**

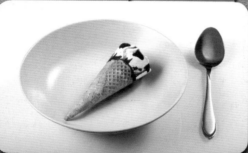

Weight: 73g

Panna Cotta

25g CARBS | **415 CALS**

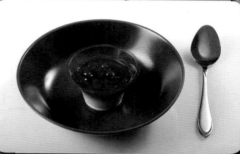

Weight: 145g

Ice Cream Lolly

26g CARBS | **267 CALS**

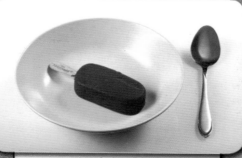

Weight: 89g

Strawberry Tartlet

35g CARBS | **272 CALS**

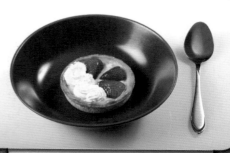

Weight: 132g

Jelly

10g CARBS **40 CALS**

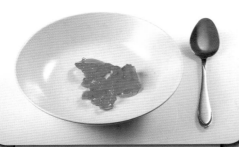

Weight: 65g

20g CARBS **79 CALS**

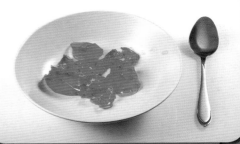

Weight: 130g

30g CARBS **122 CALS**

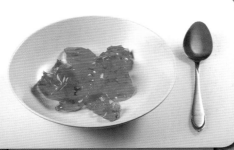

Weight: 200g

40g CARBS **162 CALS**

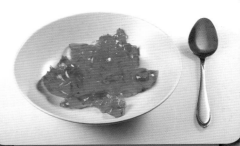

Weight: 265g

50g CARBS **201 CALS**

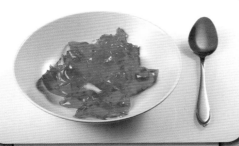

Weight: 330g

60g CARBS **244 CALS**

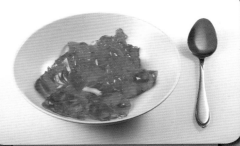

Weight: 400g

Lemon Meringue Pie

19g CARBS **110 CALS**

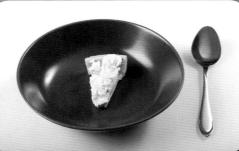

Weight: 44g

38g CARBS **221 CALS**

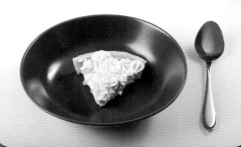

Weight: 88g

57g CARBS **326 CALS**

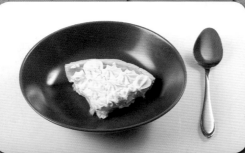

Weight: 130g

76g CARBS **439 CALS**

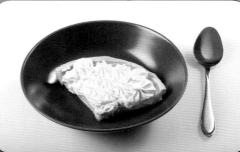

Weight: 175g

95g CARBS **547 CALS**

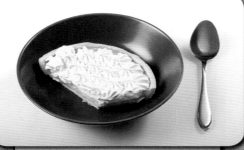

Weight: 218g

114g CARBS **658 CALS**

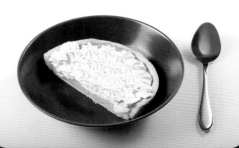

Weight: 262g

Mousse (chocolate)

10g CARBS **75 CALS**

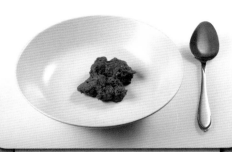

Weight: 50g

20g CARBS **149 CALS**

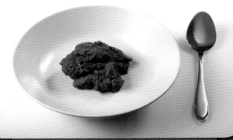

Weight: 100g

30g CARBS **224 CALS**

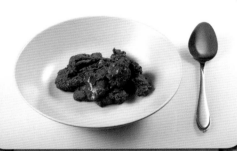

Weight: 150g

40g CARBS **298 CALS**

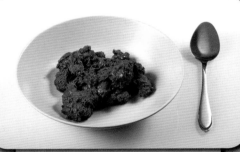

Weight: 200g

50g CARBS **373 CALS**

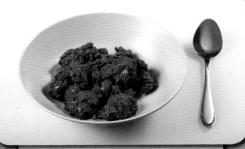

Weight: 250g

60g CARBS **447 CALS**

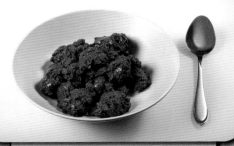

Weight: 300g

Profiteroles

10g CARBS | 138 CALS

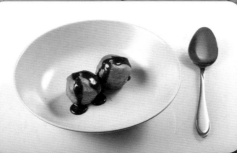

Weight: 40g

20g CARBS | 277 CALS

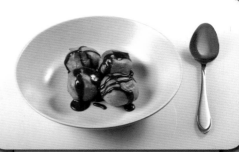

Weight: 80g

30g CARBS | 415 CALS

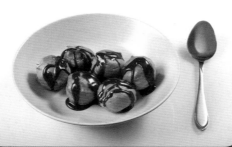

Weight: 120g

40g CARBS | 557 CALS

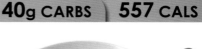
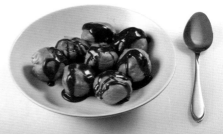

Weight: 161g

50g CARBS | 709 CALS

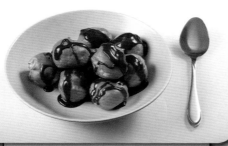

Weight: 205g

60g CARBS | 848 CALS

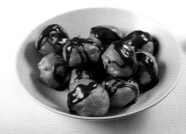

Weight: 245g

Rice Pudding

11g CARBS — **60 CALS**

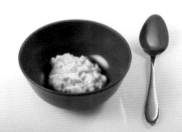

Weight: 70g

23g CARBS — **119 CALS**

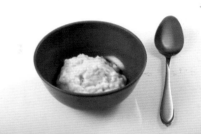

Weight: 140g

35g CARBS — **183 CALS**

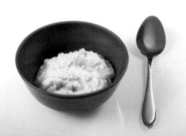

Weight: 215g

46g CARBS — **242 CALS**

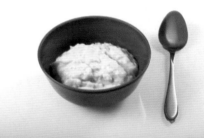

Weight: 285g

57g CARBS — **302 CALS**

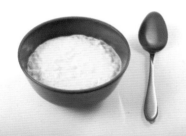

Weight: 355g

68g CARBS — **361 CALS**

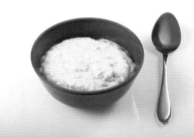

Weight: 425g

Roulade

18g CARBS | **154 CALS**

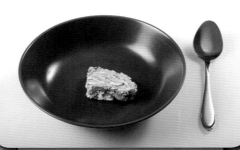

Weight: 38g

36g CARBS | **308 CALS**

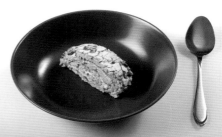

Weight: 76g

54g CARBS | **462 CALS**

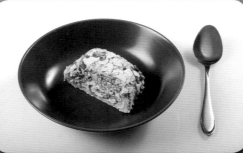

Weight: 114g

72g CARBS | **624 CALS**

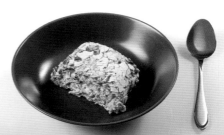

Weight: 154g

90g CARBS | **778 CALS**

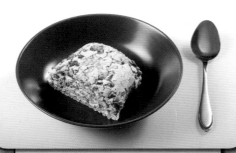

Weight: 192g

108g CARBS | **932 CALS**

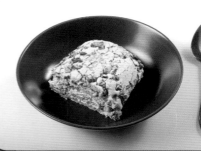

Weight: 230g

Spotted Dick

25g CARBS   **180 CALS**

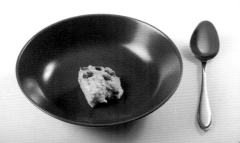

Weight: 52g

50g CARBS   **363 CALS**

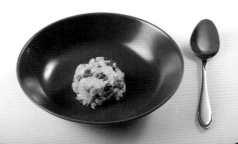

Weight: 105g (individual)

75g CARBS   **547 CALS**

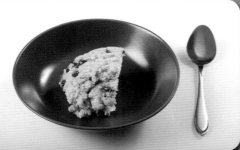

Weight: 158g

100g CARBS   **730 CALS**

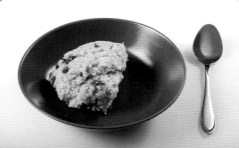

Weight: 211g

125g CARBS   **913 CALS**

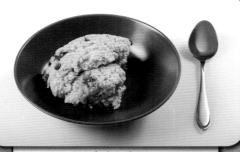

Weight: 264g

150g CARBS   **1097 CALS**

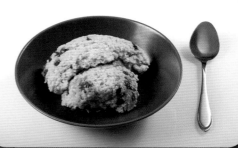

Weight: 317g

Sticky Toffee Pudding

13g CARBS   **103 CALS**

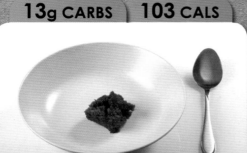

Weight: 31g

26g CARBS   **205 CALS**

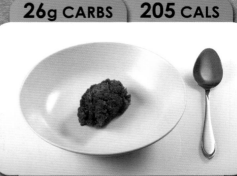

Weight: 62g

39g CARBS   **311 CALS**

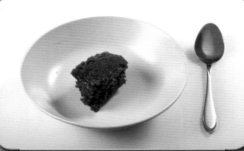

Weight: 94g

52g CARBS   **414 CALS**

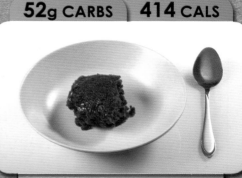

Weight: 125g

65g CARBS   **523 CALS**

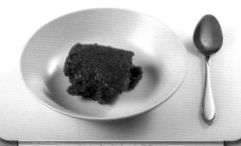

Weight: 158g

78g CARBS   **626 CALS**

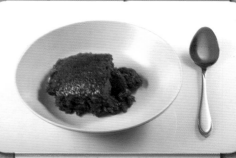

Weight: 189g

Strawberry Delight

5g CARBS | **38 CALS**

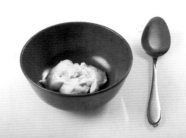

Weight: 33g

15g CARBS | **116 CALS**

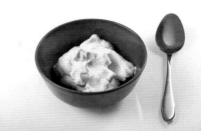

Weight: 100g

25g CARBS | **193 CALS**

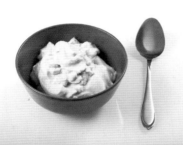

Weight: 166g

35g CARBS | **270 CALS**

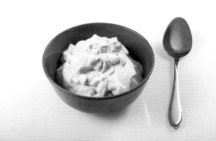

Weight: 233g

45g CARBS | **348 CALS**

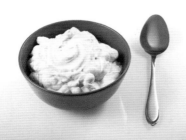

Weight: 300g

56g CARBS | **427 CALS**

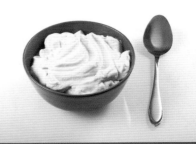

Weight: 368g

Summer Pudding

10g CARBS   **43 CALS**

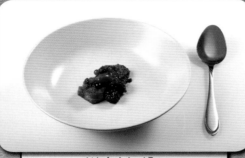

Weight: 45g

20g CARBS   **89 CALS**

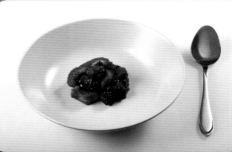

Weight: 94g

30g CARBS   **133 CALS**

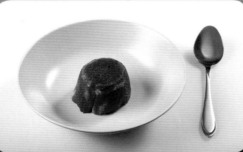

Weight: 140g (individual)

39g CARBS   **176 CALS**

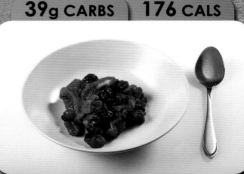

Weight: 185g

49g CARBS   **221 CALS**

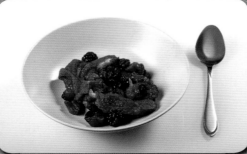

Weight: 233g

59g CARBS   **266 CALS**

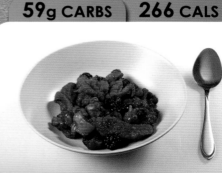

Weight: 280g

Tiramisu

15g CARBS   **119 CALS**

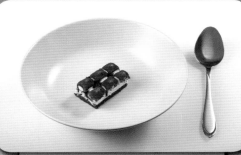

Weight: 45g

30g CARBS   **239 CALS**

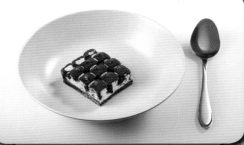

Weight: 90g

45g CARBS   **355 CALS**

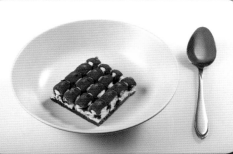

Weight: 134g

59g CARBS   **472 CALS**

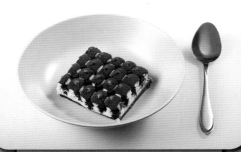

Weight: 178g

74g CARBS   **588 CALS**

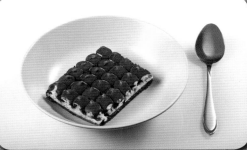

Weight: 222g

89g CARBS   **702 CALS**

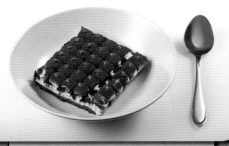

Weight: 265g

Trifle

12g CARBS   **91 CALS**

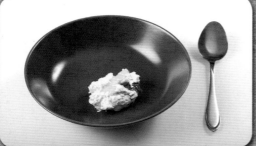

Weight: 55g

23g CARBS   **178 CALS**

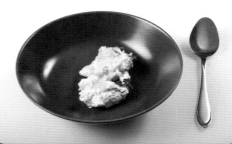

Weight: 108g

34g CARBS   **267 CALS**

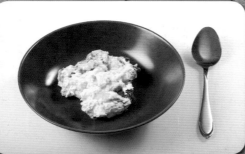

Weight: 162g

45g CARBS   **355 CALS**

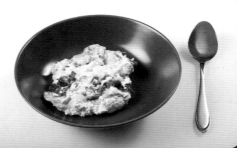

Weight: 215g

57g CARBS   **446 CALS**

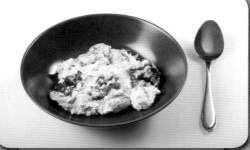

Weight: 270g

68g CARBS   **536 CALS**

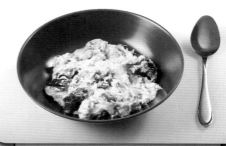

Weight: 325g

Apple Juice

| 16g CARBS | 28g CARBS | 57g CARBS |
| 61 CALS | 109 CALS | 218 CALS |

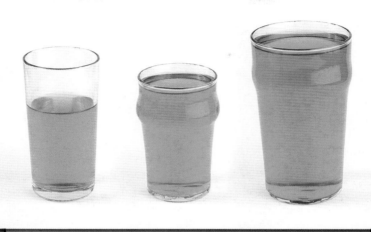

| 160ml | 284ml (half pint) | 568ml (pint) |

Cranberry Juice

| 23g CARBS | 41g CARBS | 83g CARBS |
| 98 CALS | 175 CALS | 350 CALS |

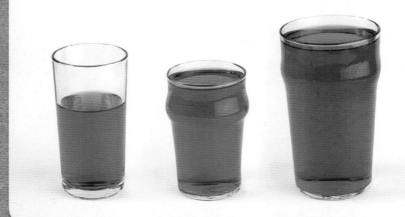

| 160ml | 284ml (half pint) | 568ml (pint) |

Grapefruit Juice

| 13g CARBS | 24g CARBS | 48g CARBS |
| 53 CALS | 95 CALS | 189 CALS |

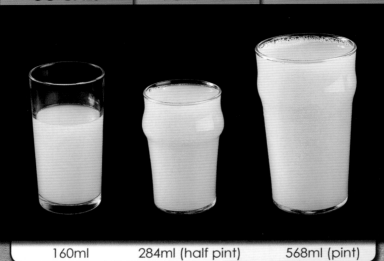

| 160ml | 284ml (half pint) | 568ml (pint) |

Orange Juice

| 14g CARBS | 25g CARBS | 51g CARBS |
| 58 CALS | 103 CALS | 207 CALS |

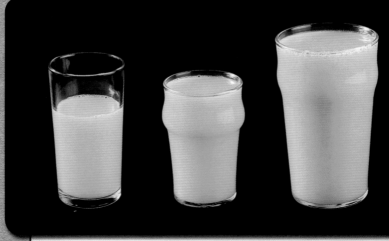

| 160ml | 284ml (half pint) | 568ml (pint) |

Pineapple Juice

17g CARBS	30g CARBS	60g CARBS
66 CALS	118 CALS	235 CALS

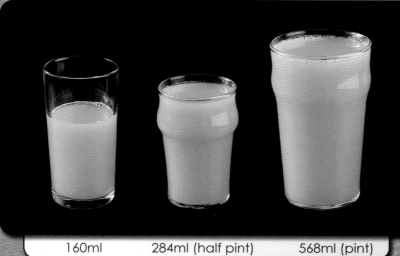

| 160ml | 284ml (half pint) | 568ml (pint) |

Tomato Juice

5g CARBS	9g CARBS	17g CARBS
22 CALS	40 CALS	80 CALS

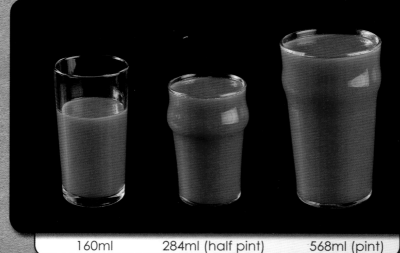

| 160ml | 284ml (half pint) | 568ml (pint) |

Cola

| 17g CARBS | 31g CARBS | 63g CARBS |
| 66 CALS | 118 CALS | 235 CALS |

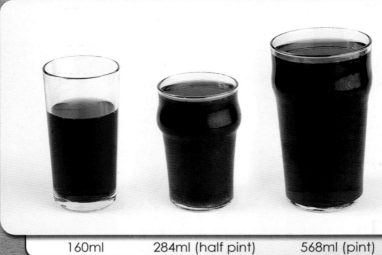

| 160ml | 284ml (half pint) | 568ml (pint) |

Lucozade Energy

| 10g CARBS | 20g CARBS | 30g CARBS |
| 39 CALS | 80 CALS | 119 CALS |

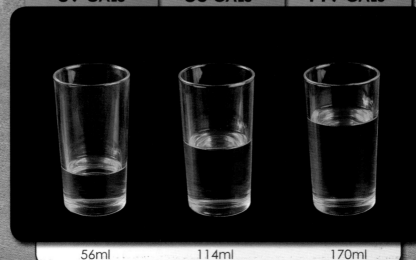

| 56ml | 114ml | 170ml |

Milk (skimmed)

7g CARBS	13g CARBS	25g CARBS
51 CALS	92 CALS	184 CALS

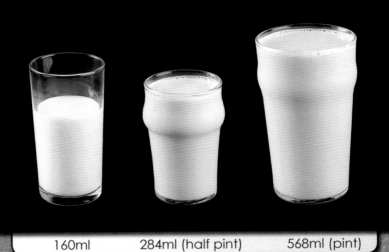

160ml	284ml (half pint)	568ml (pint)

Milk (semi-skimmed)

8g CARBS	13g CARBS	27g CARBS
74 CALS	132 CALS	264 CALS

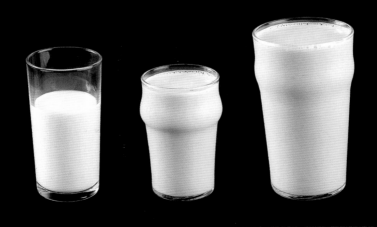

160ml	284ml (half pint)	568ml (pint)

Milk (whole)

7g CARBS	13g CARBS	26g CARBS
106 CALS	189 CALS	379 CALS

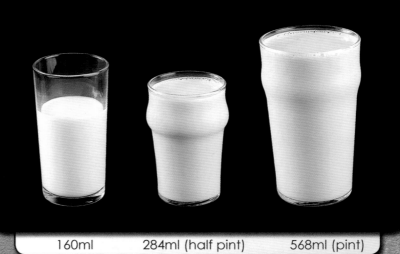

| 160ml | 284ml (half pint) | 568ml (pint) |

Soya Milk (sweetened)

4g CARBS	7g CARBS	14g CARBS
69 CALS	123 CALS	247 CALS

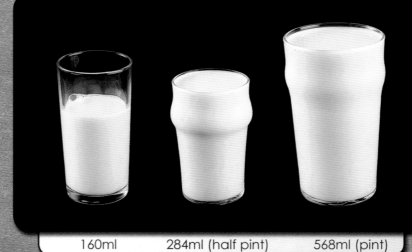

| 160ml | 284ml (half pint) | 568ml (pint) |

Fruit Smoothie (strawberry & banana)

20g CARBS	84 CALS	73g CARBS	302 CALS

160ml

568ml (pint)

Milkshake (made with powder & semi-skimmed milk)

32g CARBS	198 CALS	65g CARBS	396 CALS

284ml (half pint)

568ml (pint)

Hot Chocolate

Hot Malt Drink

28g CARBS	190 CALS	34g CARBS	221 CALS

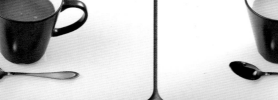

260ml

260ml

* SEE PAGE 10

Lager (draught) *

4g CARBS | **95 CALS**

284ml (half pint)

8g CARBS | **189 CALS**

568ml (pint)

Ale *

9g CARBS | **86 CALS**

284ml (half pint)

17g CARBS | **172 CALS**

568ml (pint)

Stout *

4g CARBS | **86 CALS**

284ml (half pint)

9g CARBS | **172 CALS**

568ml (pint)

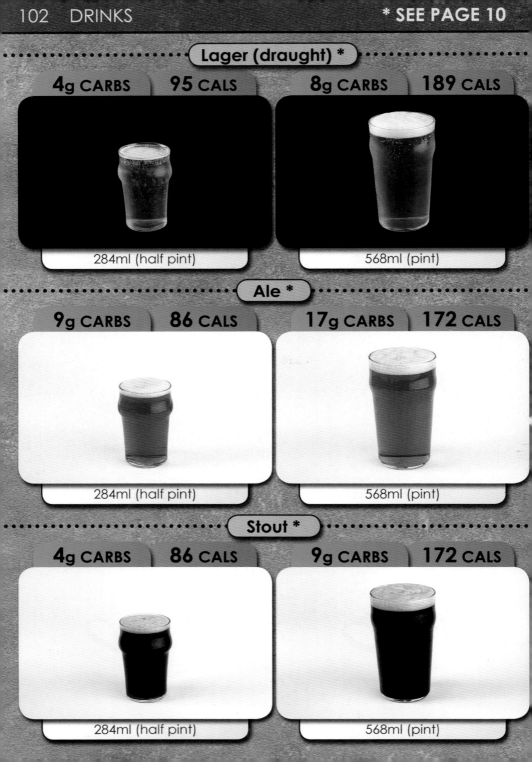

Cider (dry) *

7g CARBS   **103 CALS**

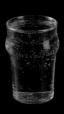

284ml (half pint)

15g CARBS   **207 CALS**

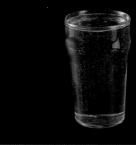

568ml (pint)

Cider (sweet) *

12g CARBS   **121 CALS**

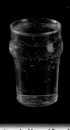

284ml (half pint)

25g CARBS   **241 CALS**

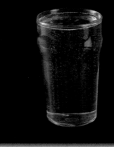

568ml (pint)

Cider (vintage) *

21g CARBS   **290 CALS**

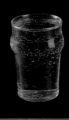

284ml (half pint)

42g CARBS   **580 CALS**

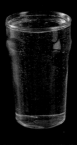

568ml (pint)

* SEE PAGE 10

Sweet White Wine *

7g CARBS **118 CALS**

125ml (small glass)

15g CARBS **235 CALS**

250ml (large glass)

Advocaat *

14g CARBS **130 CALS**

50ml

Vermouth (sweet) *

8g CARBS **76 CALS**

50ml

Port *

6g CARBS **79 CALS**

50ml

Sweet Liqueur *

8g CARBS **64 CALS**

25ml

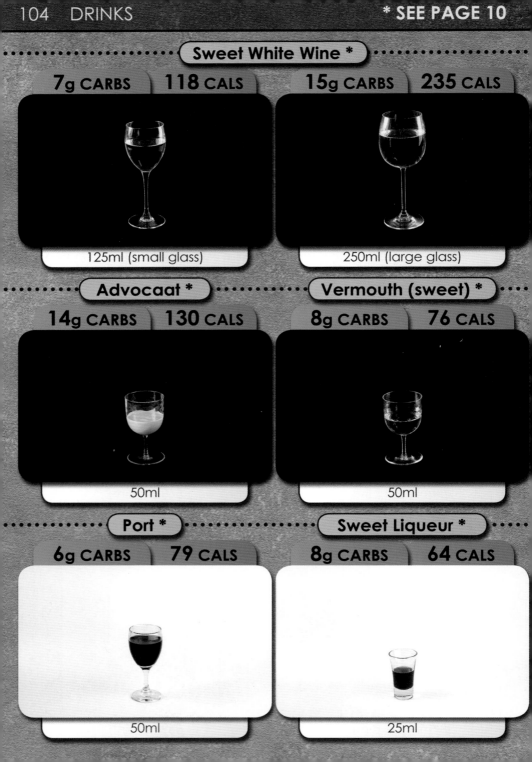

WKD *

35g CARBS   **207 CALS**

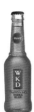

	CARBS	CALS
2x	70g	414
3x	105g	621
4x	140g	828
275ml bottle		

WKD Core (cider) *

47g CARBS   **325 CALS**

	CARBS	CALS
2x	94g	650
3x	141g	975
4x	188g	1300
500ml bottle		

Energy Drink

13g CARBS   **27g CARBS**
55 CALS   **111 CALS**

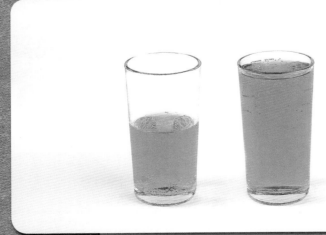

125ml (half can)   250ml (full can)

Apricot (fresh)

4g CARBS   **17 CALS**

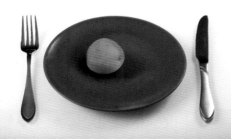

Weight: 55g

8g CARBS   **34 CALS**

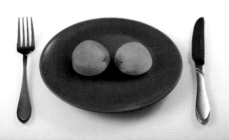

Weight: 110g

12g CARBS   **51 CALS**

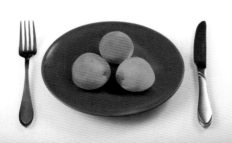

Weight: 165g

Apricot (dried)

10g CARBS   **44 CALS**

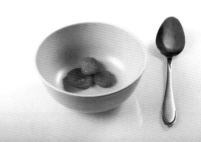

Weight: 28g

20g CARBS   **87 CALS**

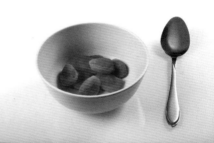

Weight: 55g

30g CARBS   **130 CALS**

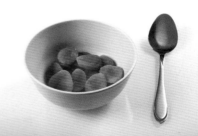

Weight: 82g

Apple

10g CARBS **40 CALS**

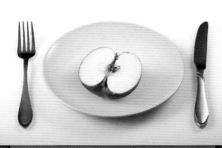

Weight: 85g

15g CARBS **62 CALS**

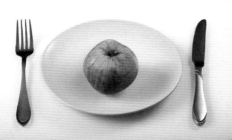

Weight: 131g

20g CARBS **80 CALS**

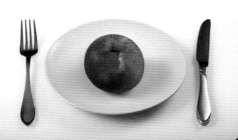

Weight: 170g

Blueberries

5g CARBS **21 CALS**

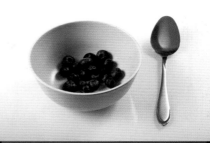

Weight: 40g

16g CARBS **69 CALS**

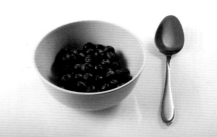

Weight: 130g

27g CARBS **114 CALS**

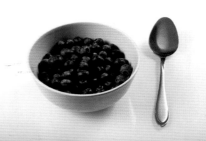

Weight: 215g

Banana

15g CARBS   **60 CALS**

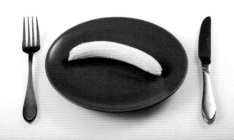

Weight: 63g (without skin)

15g CARBS   **60 CALS**

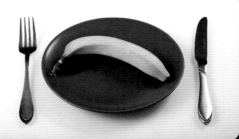

Weight: 97g (with skin)

20g CARBS   **81 CALS**

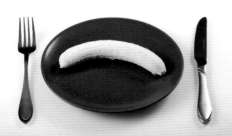

Weight: 85g (without skin)

20g CARBS   **81 CALS**

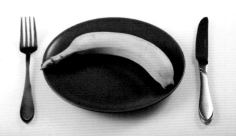

Weight: 130g (with skin)

30g CARBS   **122 CALS**

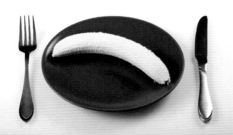

Weight: 128g (without skin)

30g CARBS   **122 CALS**

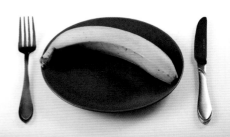

Weight: 190g (with skin)

Cherries

6g CARBS **24 CALS**

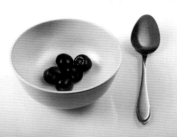

Weight: 50g (with stones)

12g CARBS **48 CALS**

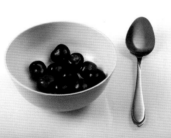

Weight: 100g (with stones)

18g CARBS **77 CALS**

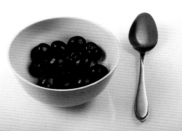

Weight: 160g (with stones)

Clementine

5g CARBS **22 CALS**

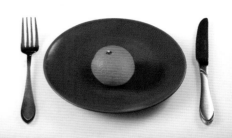

Weight: 80g

10g CARBS **45 CALS**

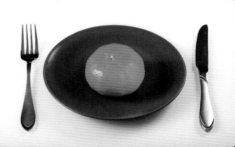

Weight: 160g

Satsuma

5g CARBS **22 CALS**

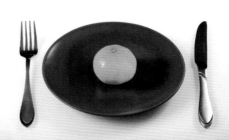

Weight: 85g

Fruit Cocktail (in juice)   ## Grapefruit

5g CARBS   **22 CALS**   **5g CARBS**   **24 CALS**

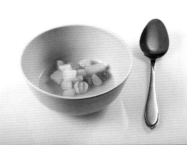   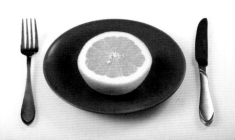

Weight: 75g   Weight: 119g (half)

15g CARBS   **61 CALS**   **10g CARBS**   **46 CALS**

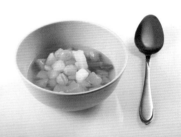   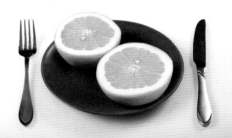

Weight: 210g (half tin)   Weight: 228g (whole)

30g CARBS   **122 CALS**   **10g CARBS**   **46 CALS**

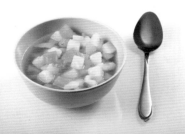   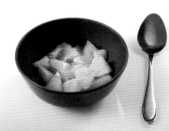

Weight: 420g (full tin)   Weight: 140g (whole)

Grapes (seedless)

10g CARBS · **39 CALS**

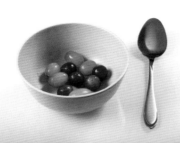

Weight: 65g

20g CARBS · **78 CALS**

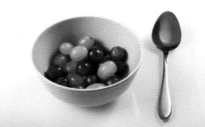

Weight: 130g

30g CARBS · **117 CALS**

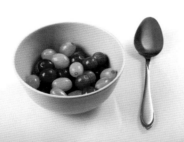

Weight: 195g

40g CARBS · **156 CALS**

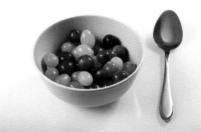

Weight: 260g

50g CARBS · **195 CALS**

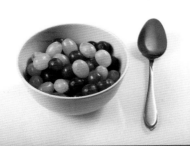

Weight: 325g

60g CARBS · **234 CALS**

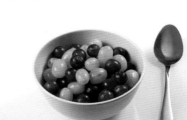

Weight: 390g

Kiwi

5g CARBS   **24 CALS**

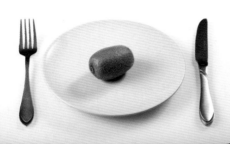

Weight: 55g (1 kiwi with skin)

5g CARBS   **24 CALS**

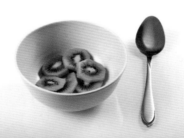

Weight: 51g (1 kiwi)

10g CARBS   **47 CALS**

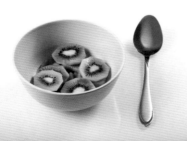

Weight: 95g (2 kiwis)

Mango

10g CARBS   **40 CALS**

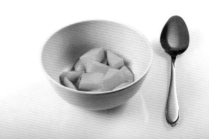

Weight: 70g

20g CARBS   **80 CALS**

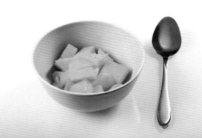

Weight: 140g

30g CARBS   **120 CALS**

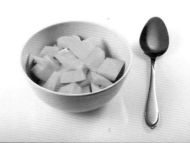

Weight: 210g

Melon (honeydew)

10g CARBS   **42 CALS**

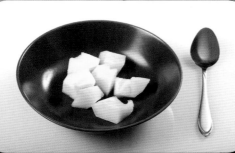

Weight: 150g

20g CARBS   **84 CALS**

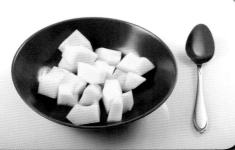

Weight: 300g

30g CARBS   **126 CALS**

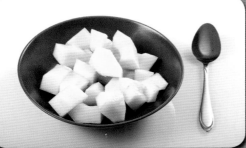

Weight: 450g

Watermelon

10g CARBS   **43 CALS**

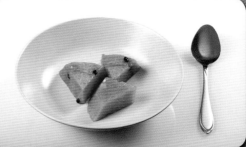

Weight: 140g

20g CARBS   **87 CALS**

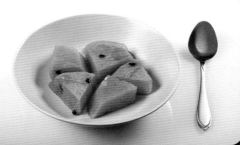

Weight: 280g

30g CARBS   **130 CALS**

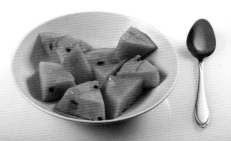

Weight: 420g

Orange

Papaya

4g CARBS   **18 CALS**   **5g CARBS**   **24 CALS**

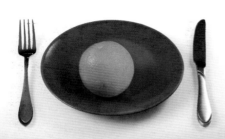

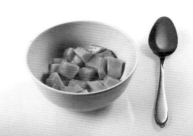

Weight: 71g   Weight: 90g

7g CARBS   **30 CALS**   **10g CARBS**   **49 CALS**

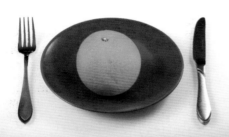

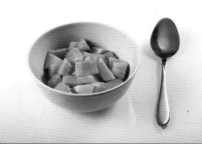

Weight: 115g   Weight: 180g

10g CARBS   **45 CALS**   **15g CARBS**   **73 CALS**

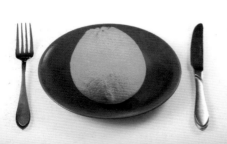

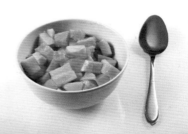

Weight: 172g   Weight: 270g

Peach (fresh)

5g CARBS | **23 CALS**

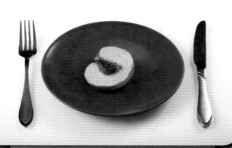

Weight: 70g (without stone)

10g CARBS | **46 CALS**

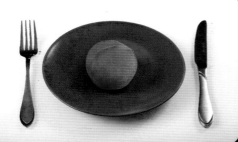

Weight: 138g

15g CARBS | **66 CALS**

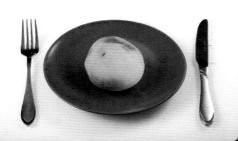

Weight: 200g

Peach (tinned in juice)

10g CARBS | **39 CALS**

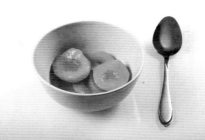

Weight: 100g

20g CARBS | **80 CALS**

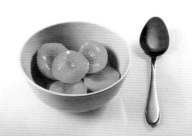

Weight: 205g (half tin)

40g CARBS | **160 CALS**

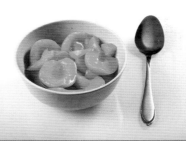

Weight: 410g (full tin)

Pear

10g CARBS   **42 CALS**

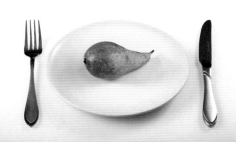

Weight: 104g

20g CARBS   **78 CALS**

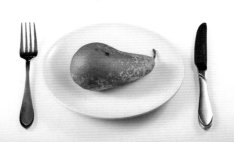

Weight: 195g

30g CARBS   **118 CALS**

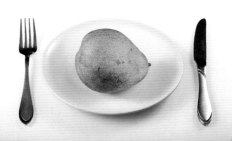

Weight: 295g

Pear (tinned in juice)

10g CARBS   **38 CALS**

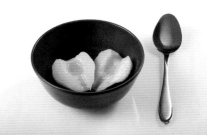

Weight: 115g

20g CARBS   **76 CALS**

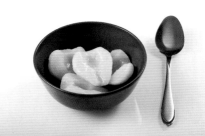

Weight: 230g

30g CARBS   **117 CALS**

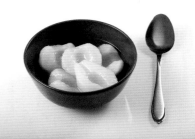

Weight: 355g (full tin)

Pineapple (fresh)

4g CARBS   **16 CALS**

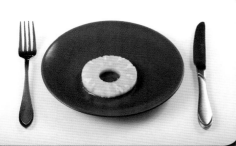

Weight: 40g

8g CARBS   **33 CALS**

Weight: 80g

12g CARBS   **49 CALS**

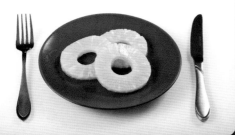

Weight: 120g

16g CARBS   **66 CALS**

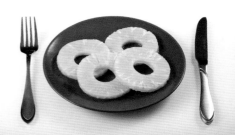

Weight: 160g

20g CARBS   **82 CALS**

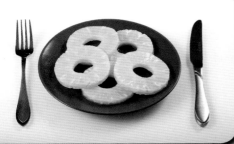

Weight: 200g

24g CARBS   **98 CALS**

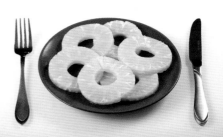

Weight: 240g

Pineapple (tinned in juice)

5g CARBS | 19 CALS
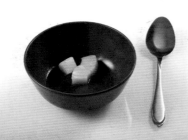
Weight: 40g

10g CARBS | 38 CALS
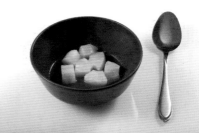
Weight: 80g

20g CARBS | 75 CALS
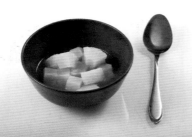
Weight: 160g

30g CARBS | 115 CALS
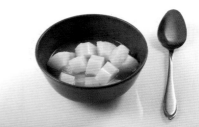
Weight: 245g

40g CARBS | 155 CALS
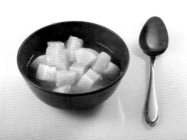
Weight: 330g

50g CARBS | 193 CALS
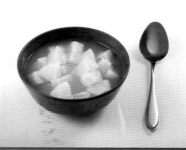
Weight: 410g (full tin)

Pomegranate

5g CARBS   **20** CALS

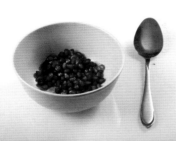

Weight: 40g

10g CARBS   **43** CALS

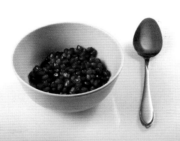

Weight: 85g

15g CARBS   **64** CALS

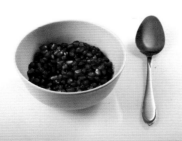

Weight: 125g

Prune

10g CARBS   **42** CALS

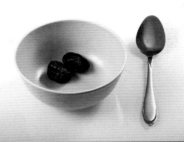

Weight: 30g

20g CARBS   **85** CALS

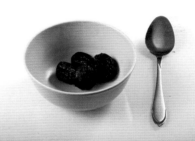

Weight: 60g

30g CARBS   **125** CALS

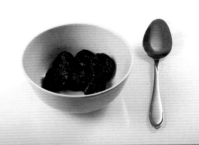

Weight: 89g

Plum

5g CARBS · 20 CALS

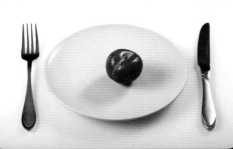

	CARBS	CALS
2x	10g	40
3x	15g	60
4x	20g	80
Weight: 55g		

10g CARBS · 40 CALS

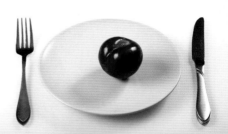

	CARBS	CALS
2x	20g	80
3x	30g	120
4x	40g	160
Weight: 110g		

Nectarine

7g CARBS · 32 CALS

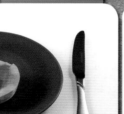

	CARBS	CALS
2x	14g	64
3x	21g	96
4x	28g	128
Weight: 80g (without stone)		

15g CARBS · 66 CALS

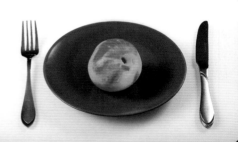

	CARBS	CALS
2x	30g	132
3x	45g	198
4x	60g	264
Weight: 165g		

Raspberries

5g CARBS   **26** CALS

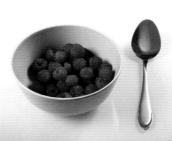

Weight: 105g

10g CARBS   **53** CALS

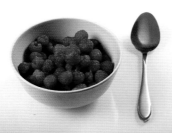

Weight: 210g

15g CARBS   **80** CALS

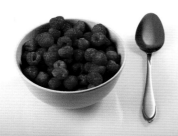

Weight: 320g

Strawberries

5g CARBS   **23** CALS

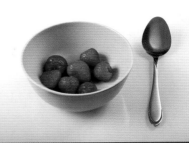

Weight: 85g

15g CARBS   **68** CALS

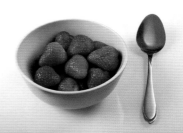

Weight: 250g

25g CARBS   **111** CALS

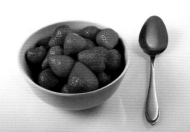

Weight: 410g

Raisins

10g CARBS   **41 CALS**

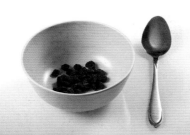

Weight: 15g

20g CARBS   **79 CALS**

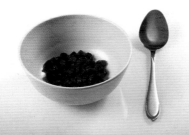

Weight: 29g

30g CARBS   **120 CALS**

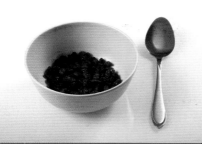

Weight: 44g

Sultanas

10g CARBS   **41 CALS**

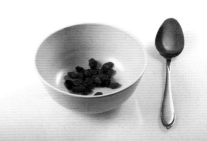

Weight: 15g

20g CARBS   **80 CALS**

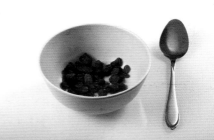

Weight: 29g

30g CARBS   **118 CALS**

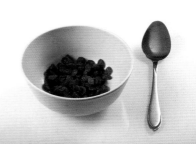

Weight: 43g

Beans on Toast (with margarine)

22g CARBS   **151 CALS**

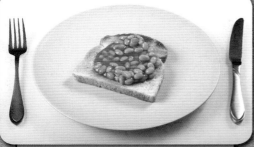

22g toast, 65g beans, 5g marg

32g CARBS   **205 CALS**

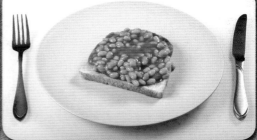

22g toast, 130g beans, 5g marg

42g CARBS   **260 CALS**

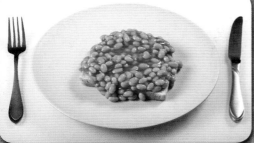

22g toast, 195g beans, 5g marg

55g CARBS   **356 CALS**

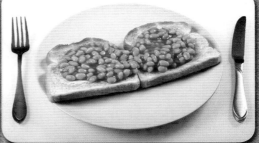

44g toast, 195g beans, 10g marg

70g CARBS   **438 CALS**

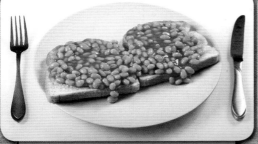

44g toast, 293g beans, 10g marg

85g CARBS   **520 CALS**

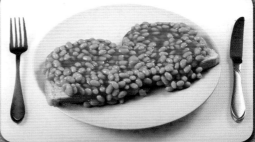

44g toast, 390g beans, 10g marg

Chicken Goujons, Potato Faces & Peas

18g CARBS **172 CALS**

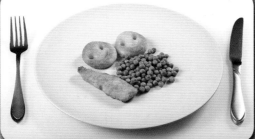

30g chick, 34g faces, 25g peas

38g CARBS **346 CALS**

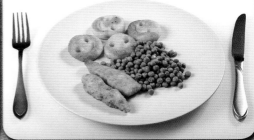

60g chick, 68g faces, 50g peas

56g CARBS **518 CALS**

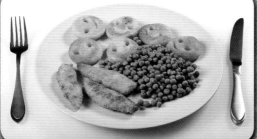

90g chick, 102g faces, 75g peas

76g CARBS **691 CALS**

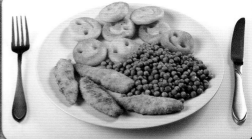

120g chick, 136g faces, 100g peas

93g CARBS **864 CALS**

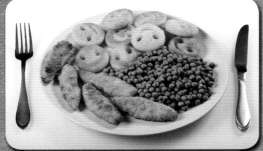

150g chick, 170g faces, 125g peas

113g CARBS **1038 CALS**

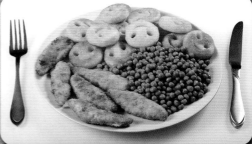

180g chick, 204g faces, 150g peas

Chilli con Carne with White Rice

15g CARBS | **137 CALS**

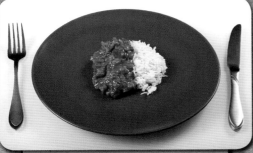

90g chilli, 32g rice

40g CARBS | **307 CALS**

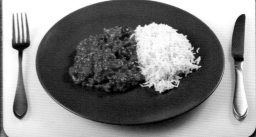

170g chilli, 96g rice

65g CARBS | **483 CALS**

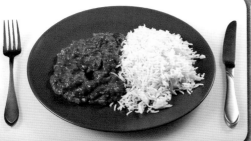

250g chilli, 163g rice

91g CARBS | **661 CALS**

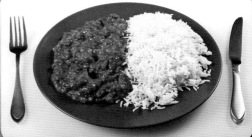

340g chilli, 225g rice

116g CARBS | **843 CALS**

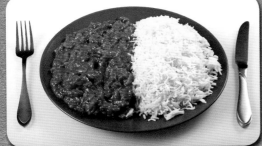

430g chilli, 290g rice

141g CARBS | **1015 CALS**

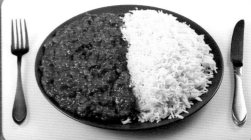

510g chilli, 355g rice

Corned Beef Hash

12g CARBS | **141 CALS**

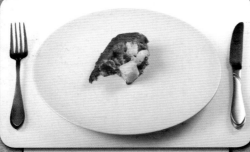

Weight: 100g

25g CARBS | **282 CALS**

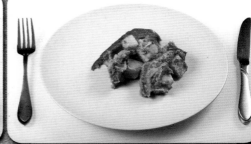

Weight: 200g

37g CARBS | **423 CALS**

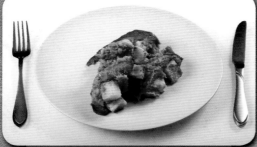

Weight: 300g

49g CARBS | **564 CALS**

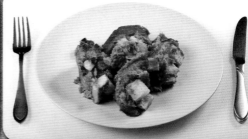

Weight: 400g

62g CARBS | **705 CALS**

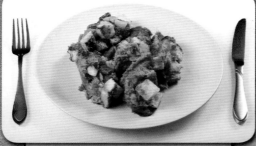

Weight: 500g

74g CARBS | **846 CALS**

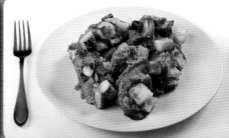

Weight: 600g

Curry (chicken) with White Rice

12g CARBS   **146 CALS**

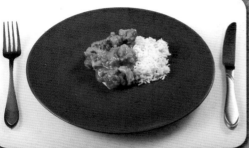

105g curry, 31g rice

35g CARBS   **390 CALS**

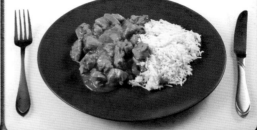

260g curry, 98g rice

57g CARBS   **580 CALS**

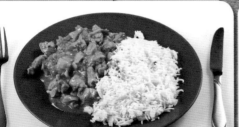

365g curry, 161g rice

79g CARBS   **810 CALS**

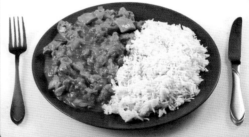

505g curry, 228g rice

101g CARBS   **1013 CALS**

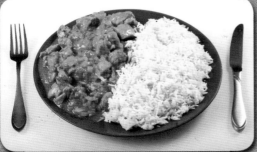

625g curry, 290g rice

124g CARBS   **1267 CALS**

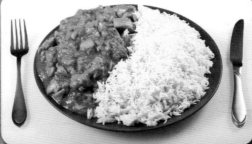

790g curry, 357g rice

Curry (lentil) with Brown Rice

20g CARBS   **179** CALS

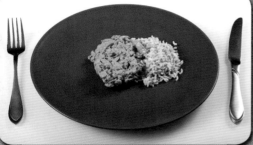

95g curry, 30g rice

49g CARBS   **400** CALS

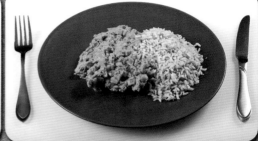

185g curry, 95g rice

79g CARBS   **624** CALS

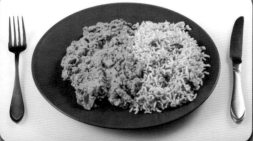

280g curry, 157g rice

110g CARBS   **856** CALS

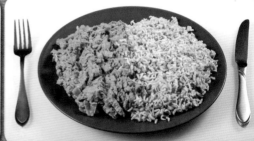

380g curry, 219g rice

140g CARBS   **1080** CALS

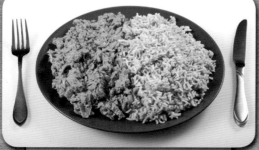

475g curry, 281g rice

170g CARBS   **1306** CALS

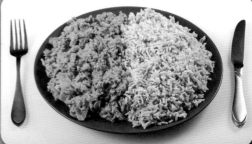

570g curry, 344g rice

Curry (veg & potato) with White Rice

20g CARBS | **120** CALS

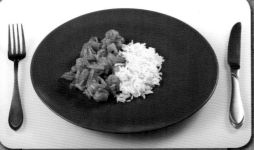

90g curry, 32g rice

49g CARBS | **281** CALS

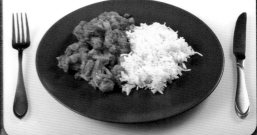

175g curry, 97g rice

78g CARBS | **443** CALS

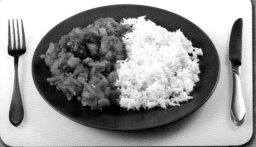

260g curry, 163g rice

108g CARBS | **607** CALS

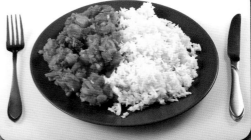

350g curry, 227g rice

138g CARBS | **772** CALS

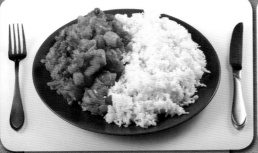

440g curry, 291g rice

167g CARBS | **935** CALS

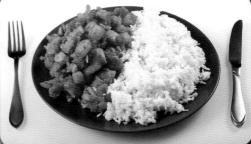

530g curry, 355g rice

Fish Fingers (grilled), Chips (oven) & Beans

30g CARBS | **185 CALS**

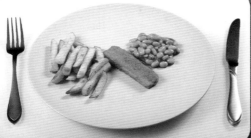

20g fish, 66g chips, 45g beans

51g CARBS | **316 CALS**

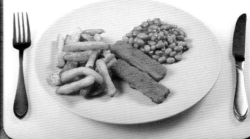

40g fish, 99g chips, 90g beans

70g CARBS | **444 CALS**

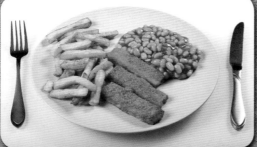

60g fish, 130g chips, 135g beans

90g CARBS | **578 CALS**

80g fish, 165g chips, 180g beans

111g CARBS | **714 CALS**

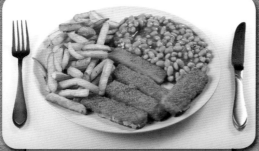

100g fish, 198g chips, 230g beans

131g CARBS | **844 CALS**

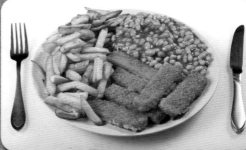

120g fish, 230g chips, 275g beans

Fish Pie

11g CARBS | **148 CALS**

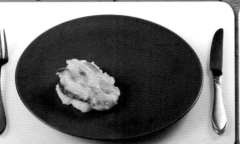

Weight: 125g

22g CARBS | **295 CALS**

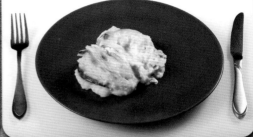

Weight: 250g

34g CARBS | **448 CALS**

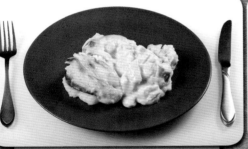

Weight: 380g

45g CARBS | **596 CALS**

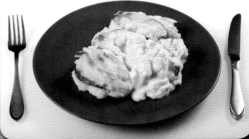

Weight: 505g

56g CARBS | **743 CALS**

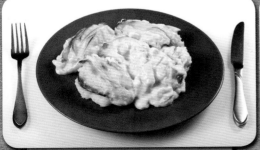

Weight: 630g

68g CARBS | **897 CALS**

Weight: 760g

Lasagne

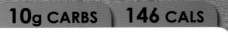

10g CARBS | **146 CALS**

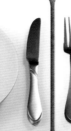

Weight: 80g

25g CARBS | **357 CALS**

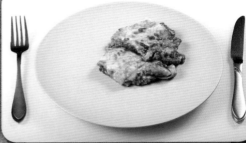

Weight: 195g

40g CARBS | **576 CALS**

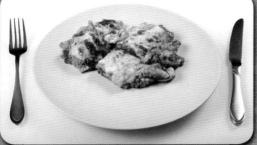

Weight: 315g

55g CARBS | **787 CALS**

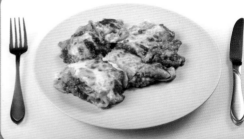

Weight: 430g

70g CARBS | **997 CALS**

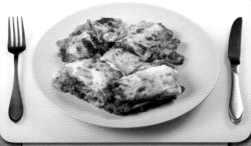

Weight: 545g

85g CARBS | **1217 CALS**

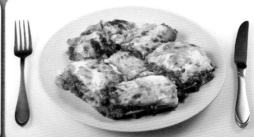

Weight: 665g

Macaroni Cheese

14g CARBS   **166 CALS**

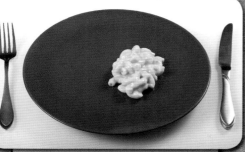

Weight: 80g

30g CARBS   **337 CALS**

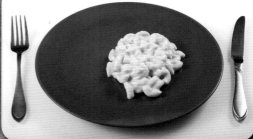

Weight: 163g

40g CARBS   **460 CALS**

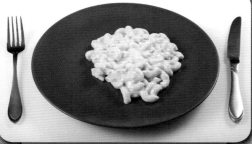

Weight: 222g

55g CARBS   **629 CALS**

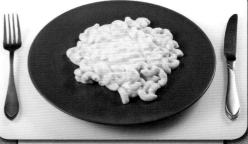

Weight: 304g

70g CARBS   **797 CALS**

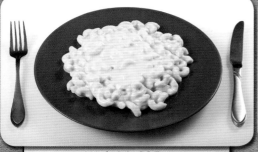

Weight: 385g

84g CARBS   **963 CALS**

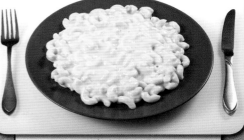

Weight: 465g

Enchilada (chicken)

29g CARBS   **323 CALS**

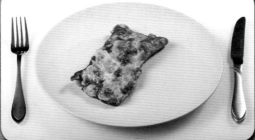

	CARBS	CALS
2x	58g	646
3x	87g	969
4x	116g	1292
Weight: 146g		

Fajita (chicken)

30g CARBS   **245 CALS**

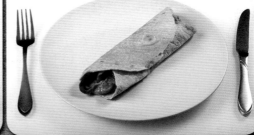

	CARBS	CALS
2x	60g	490
3x	90g	735
4x	120g	980
Weight: 160g		

Quesadilla (bean)

19g CARBS   **166 CALS**

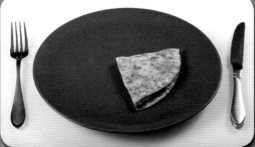

	CARBS	CALS
2x	38g	332
3x	57g	498
4x	76g	664
Weight: 74g		

Taco (beef)

10g CARBS   **238 CALS**

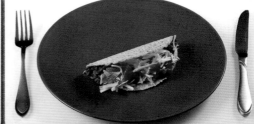

	CARBS	CALS
2x	20g	476
3x	30g	714
4x	40g	952
Weight: 80g		

Pasta Bake (tuna & cheese)

15g CARBS | **109 CALS**

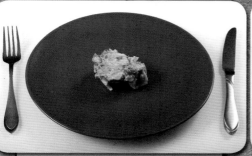

Weight: 70g

30g CARBS | **223 CALS**

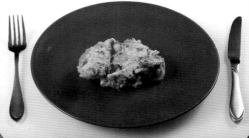

Weight: 143g

45g CARBS | **334 CALS**

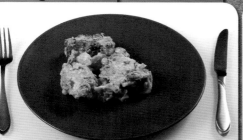

Weight: 214g

60g CARBS | **439 CALS**

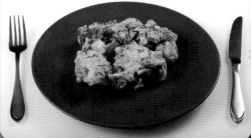

Weight: 285g

75g CARBS | **547 CALS**

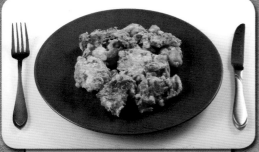

Weight: 355g

90g CARBS | **665 CALS**

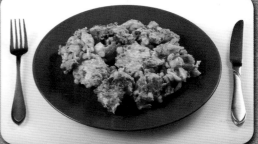

Weight: 426g

Pasta Meal (chicken & broccoli)

10g CARBS   **110 CALS**

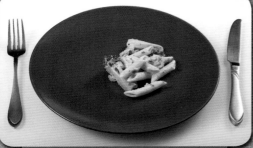

Weight: 65g

25g CARBS   **281 CALS**

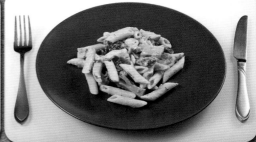

Weight: 166g

40g CARBS   **451 CALS**

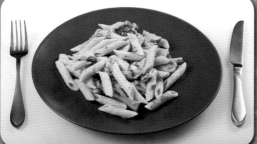

Weight: 267g

51g CARBS   **576 CALS**

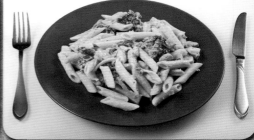

Weight: 341g

67g CARBS   **747 CALS**

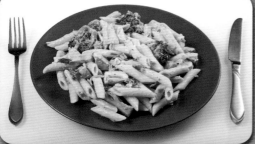

Weight: 442g

82g CARBS   **918 CALS**

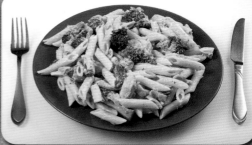

Weight: 543g

Chicken & Bacon Pie

50g CARBS | **702 CALS**

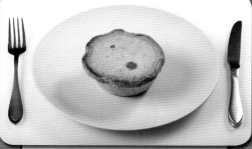

Weight: 264g

Steak Pie

56g CARBS | **632 CALS**

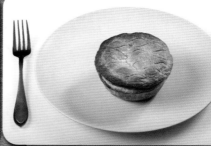

Weight: 244g

Steak & Kidney Pudding

34g CARBS | **382 CALS**

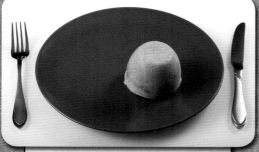

Weight: 182g

Top Crust Pie

25g CARBS | **341 CALS**

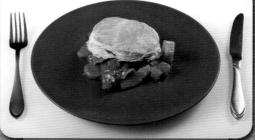

Weight: 264g

Steak & Potato Pie

25g CARBS | **307 CALS**

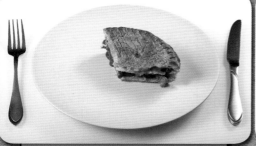

Weight: 130g

50g CARBS | **625 CALS**

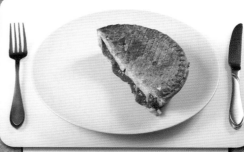

Weight: 265g

Pizza (chicken, deep pan, oven baked)

20g CARBS　143 CALS

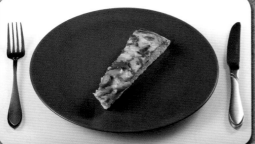

	CARBS	CALS
2x	40g	286
3x	60g	429
4x	80g	572
Weight: 65g		

40g CARBS　286 CALS

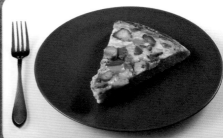

	CARBS	CALS
2x	80g	572
3x	120g	858
4x	160g	1144
Weight: 130g		

61g CARBS　429 CALS

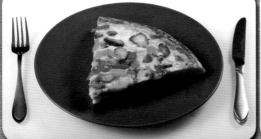

	CARBS	CALS
2x	122g	858
3x	183g	1287
4x	244g	1716
Weight: 195g		

80g CARBS　568 CALS

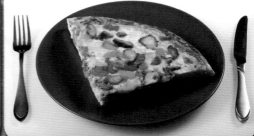

	CARBS	CALS
2x	160g	1136
3x	240g	1704
4x	320g	2272
Weight: 258g		

Pizza (pepperoni, thin crust, oven baked)

11g CARBS | **102 CALS**

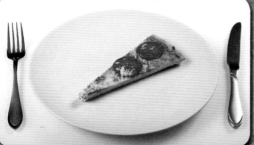

	CARBS	CALS
2x	22g	204
3x	33g	306
4x	44g	408
Weight: 40g		

20g CARBS | **191 CALS**

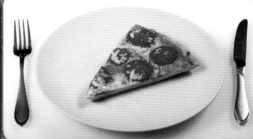

	CARBS	CALS
2x	40g	382
3x	60g	573
4x	80g	764
Weight: 75g		

30g CARBS | **293 CALS**

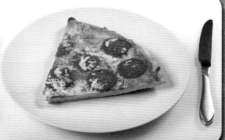

	CARBS	CALS
2x	60g	586
3x	90g	879
4x	120g	1172
Weight: 115g		

41g CARBS | **395 CALS**

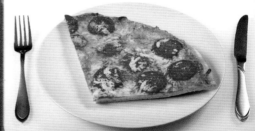

	CARBS	CALS
2x	82g	790
3x	123g	1185
4x	164g	1580
Weight: 155g		

Quiche Lorraine, Salad & Coleslaw

16g CARBS   **410 CALS**

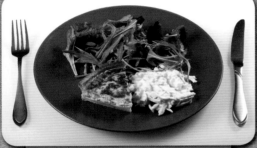

65g quiche, 65g coleslaw

29g CARBS   **668 CALS**

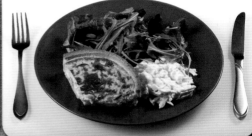

135g quiche, 65g coleslaw

44g CARBS   **1074 CALS**

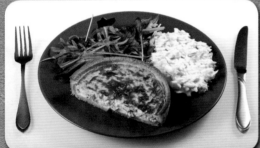

200g quiche, 130g coleslaw

57g CARBS   **1314 CALS**

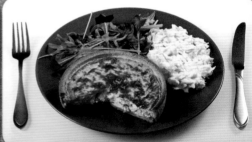

265g quiche, 130g coleslaw

73g CARBS   **1722 CALS**

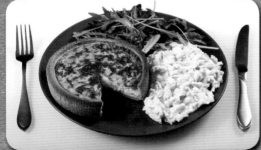

330g quiche, 195g coleslaw

86g CARBS   **1980 CALS**

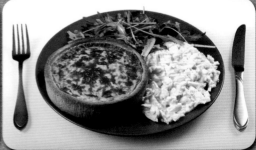

400g quiche, 195g coleslaw

Risotto (mushroom)

20g CARBS   **169** CALS
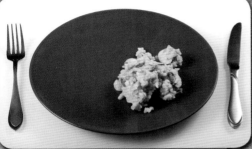
Weight: 120g

40g CARBS   **340** CALS
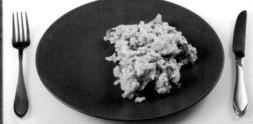
Weight: 241g

60g CARBS   **512** CALS
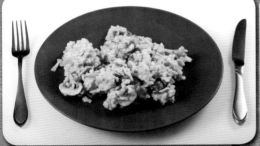
Weight: 363g

80g CARBS   **684** CALS
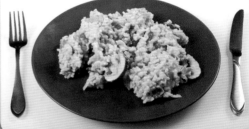
Weight: 485g

100g CARBS   **856** CALS
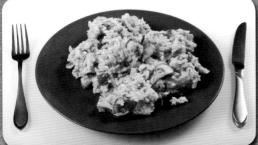
Weight: 607g

120g CARBS   **1028** CALS
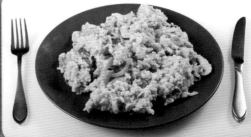
Weight: 729g

Sausage, Mash (with butter) & Onion Gravy

25g CARBS | **297 CALS**

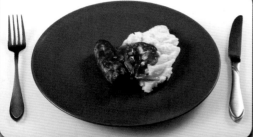

55g saus, 120g mash, 25g gravy

49g CARBS | **587 CALS**

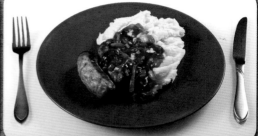

110g saus, 235g mash, 50g gravy

73g CARBS | **883 CALS**

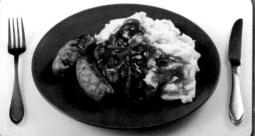

165g saus, 355g mash, 75g gravy

98g CARBS | **1175 CALS**

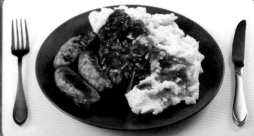

220g saus, 470g mash, 100g gravy

122g CARBS | **1472 CALS**

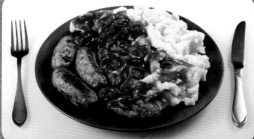

275g saus, 590g mash, 125g gravy

146g CARBS | **1762 CALS**

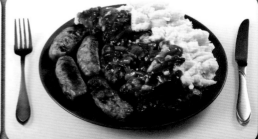

330g saus, 705g mash, 150g gravy

Shepherd's Pie

12g CARBS | **175 CALS**

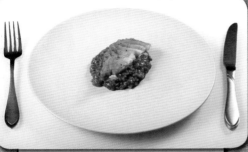

Weight: 120g

25g CARBS | **350 CALS**

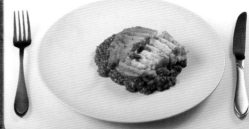

Weight: 240g

37g CARBS | **526 CALS**

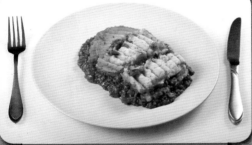

Weight: 360g

50g CARBS | **708 CALS**

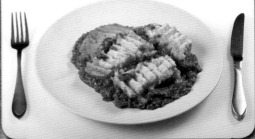

Weight: 485g

63g CARBS | **883 CALS**

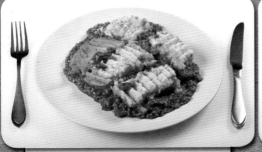

Weight: 605g

76g CARBS | **1066 CALS**

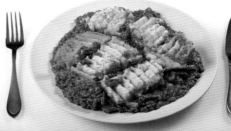

Weight: 730g

Chicken Noodle Soup

4g CARBS | **25 CALS**

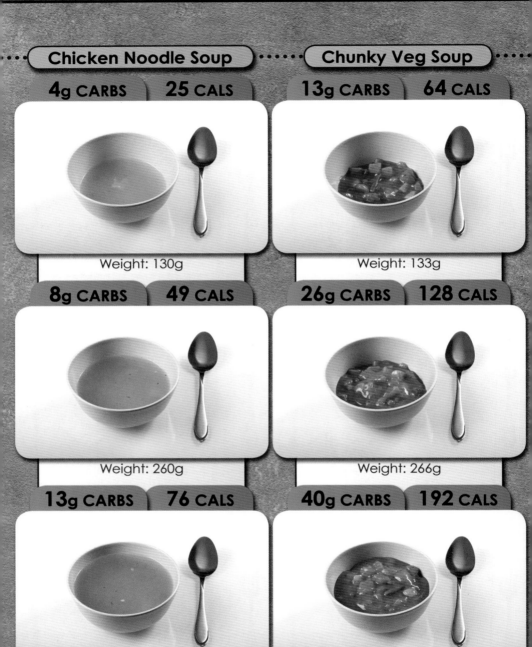

Weight: 130g

8g CARBS | **49 CALS**

Weight: 260g

13g CARBS | **76 CALS**

Weight: 400g

Chunky Veg Soup

13g CARBS | **64 CALS**

Weight: 133g

26g CARBS | **128 CALS**

Weight: 266g

40g CARBS | **192 CALS**

Weight: 400g (full tin)

Mushroom Soup

5g CARBS   **60** CALS

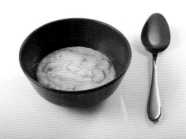

Weight: 130g

10g CARBS   **120** CALS

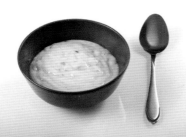

Weight: 260g

15g CARBS   **179** CALS

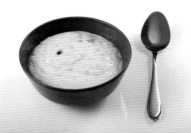

Weight: 390g (full tin)

Tomato Soup

10g CARBS   **84** CALS

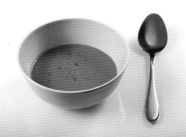

Weight: 135g

20g CARBS   **171** CALS

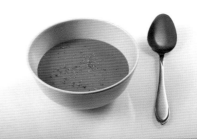

Weight: 275g

30g CARBS   **254** CALS

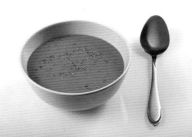

Weight: 410g (full tin)

Spaghetti Bolognese

15g CARBS   **144 CALS**

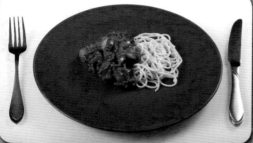

33g spag, 120g bolognese

40g CARBS   **334 CALS**

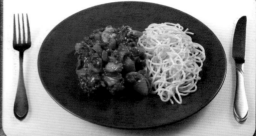

95g spag, 240g bolognese

65g CARBS   **527 CALS**

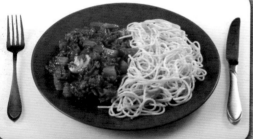

159g spag, 360g bolognese

90g CARBS   **720 CALS**

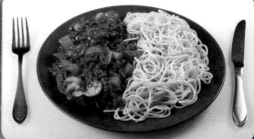

223g spag, 480g bolognese

115g CARBS   **915 CALS**

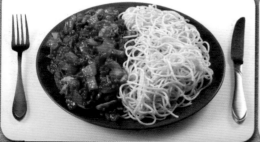

286g spag, 605g bolognese

140g CARBS   **1114 CALS**

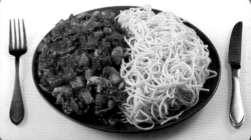

349g spag, 735g bolognese

Stew & Dumplings

20g CARBS | **204 CALS**

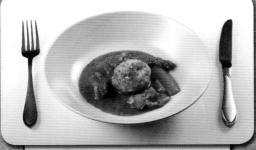

95g stew, 45g dumplings

40g CARBS | **397 CALS**

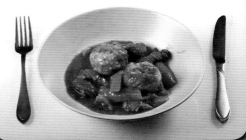

175g stew, 90g dumplings

65g CARBS | **658 CALS**

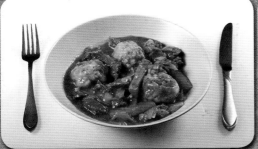

355g stew, 135g dumplings

85g CARBS | **855 CALS**

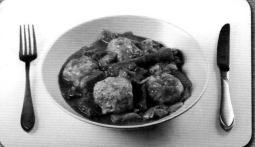

440g stew, 180g dumplings

105g CARBS | **1062 CALS**

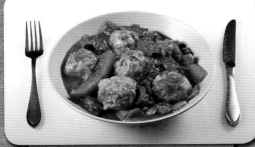

540g stew, 225g dumplings

125g CARBS | **1259 CALS**

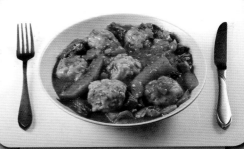

625g stew, 270g dumplings

Stir-fry (chicken)

10g CARBS   **81 CALS**

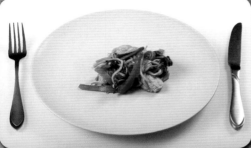

Weight: 70g

21g CARBS   **162 CALS**

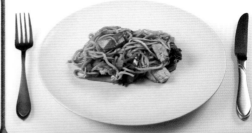

Weight: 140g

30g CARBS   **238 CALS**

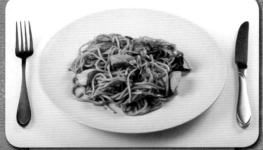

Weight: 205g

41g CARBS   **319 CALS**

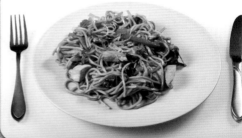

Weight: 275g

51g CARBS   **400 CALS**

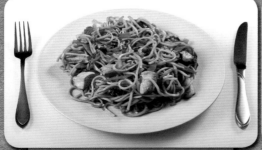

Weight: 345g

61g CARBS   **477 CALS**

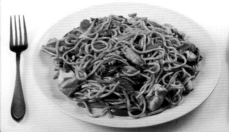

Weight: 411g

Sushi

9g CARBS   53 CALS

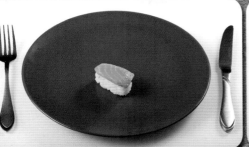

	CARBS	CALS
2x	18g	106
3x	27g	159
4x	36g	212
Weight: 34g	

10g CARBS   58 CALS

	CARBS	CALS
2x	20g	116
3x	30g	174
4x	40g	232
Weight: 36g	

8g CARBS   44 CALS

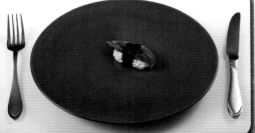

	CARBS	CALS
2x	16g	88
3x	24g	132
4x	32g	176
Weight: 28g	

6g CARBS   40 CALS

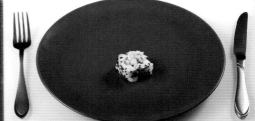

	CARBS	CALS
2x	12g	80
3x	18g	120
4x	24g	160
Weight: 24g	

Toad in the Hole

20g CARBS   **269** CALS

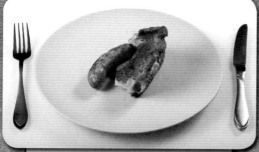

55g sausage, 37g yorkshire

40g CARBS   **534** CALS

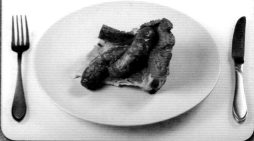

110g sausage, 73g yorkshire

60g CARBS   **803** CALS

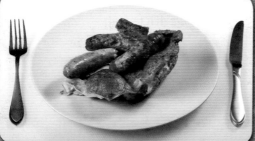

165g sausage, 110g yorkshire

80g CARBS   **1069** CALS

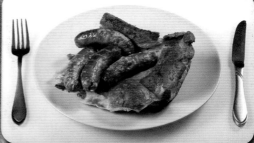

220g sausage, 146g yorkshire

100g CARBS   **1335** CALS

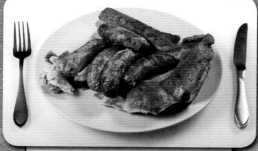

275g sausage, 182g yorkshire

119g CARBS   **1603** CALS

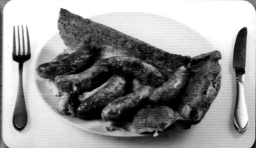

330g sausage, 219g yorkshire

Coleslaw

3g CARBS   **168 CALS**

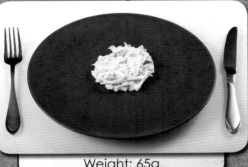

Weight: 65g

5g CARBS   **335 CALS**

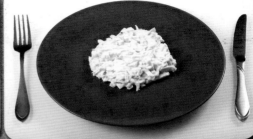

Weight: 130g

Onion Rings (battered, oven baked)

7g CARBS   **69 CALS**

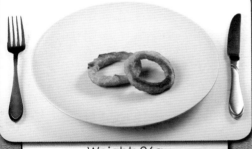

Weight: 26g

15g CARBS   **138 CALS**

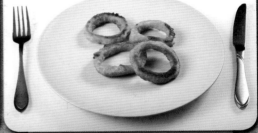

Weight: 52g

Potato Salad (with mayonnaise)

9g CARBS   **238 CALS**

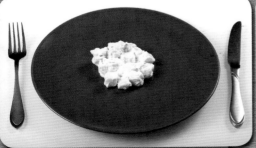

Weight: 83g

19g CARBS   **476 CALS**

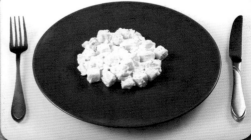

Weight: 166g

Stuffing (packet mix)

13g CARBS   **63 CALS**

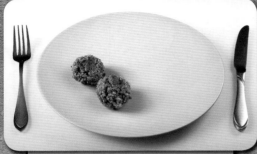

Weight: 65g

25g CARBS   **126 CALS**

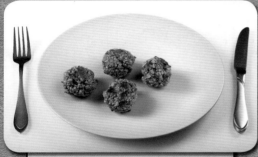

Weight: 130g

38g CARBS   **189 CALS**

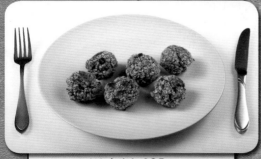

Weight: 195g

Yorkshire Pudding

10g CARBS   **84 CALS**

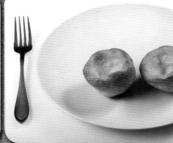

Weight: 40g

20g CARBS   **168 CALS**

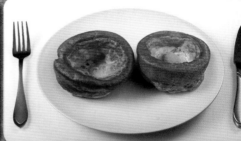

Weight: 80g

30g CARBS   **252 CALS**

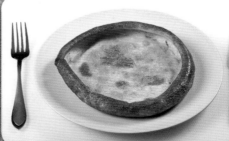

Weight: 120g

Apple Chutney

10g CARBS   **38 CALS**

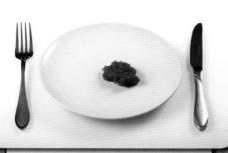

Weight: 20g

Brown Sauce

5g CARBS   **21 CALS**

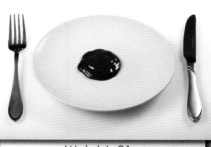

Weight: 21g

Cranberry Sauce

6g CARBS   **21 CALS**

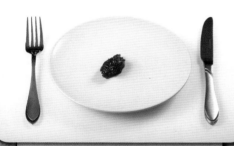

Weight: 14g

Horseradish

5g CARBS   **40 CALS**

Weight: 26g

Ketchup

5g CARBS   **22 CALS**

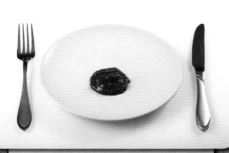

Weight: 19g

Mint Sauce

5g CARBS   **21 CALS**

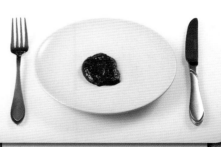

Weight: 21g

Piccalilli

4g CARBS   **18** CALS

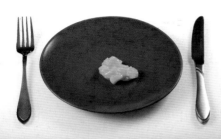

Weight: 22g

Pickle

10g CARBS   **39** CALS

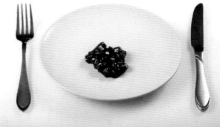

Weight: 28g

Salad Cream

5g CARBS   **94** CALS

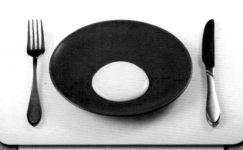

Weight: 27g

Sweet Chilli Sauce

6g CARBS   **23** CALS

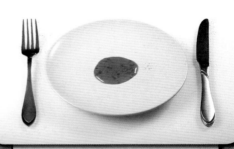

Weight: 10g

Tartar Sauce

5g CARBS   **78** CALS

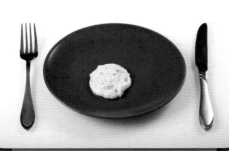

Weight: 26g

Thousand Island

5g CARBS   **116** CALS

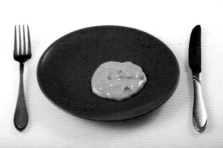

Weight: 36g

Fish (battered, baked)
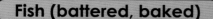

9g CARBS · **137 CALS**

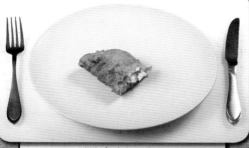

Weight: 65g

19g CARBS · **274 CALS**

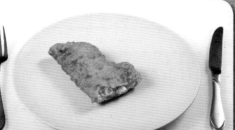

Weight: 130g

38g CARBS · **559 CALS**

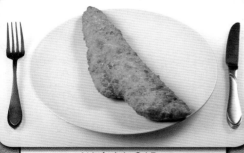

Weight: 265g

Fish (breaded, baked)
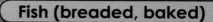

8g CARBS · **121 CALS**

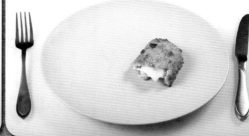

Weight: 53g

16g CARBS · **243 CALS**

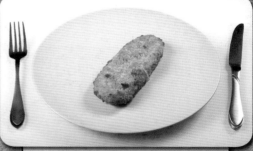

Weight: 106g

24g CARBS · **357 CALS**

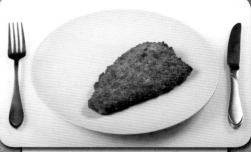

Weight: 156g

Fish Cake (baked)

10g CARBS	80 CALS

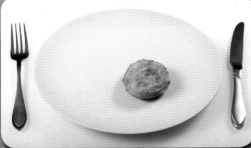

	CARBS	CALS
2x	20g	160
3x	30g	240
4x	40g	320
Weight: 52g		

18g CARBS	139 CALS

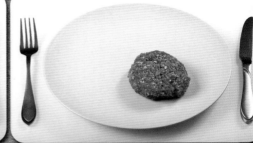

	CARBS	CALS
2x	36g	278
3x	54g	417
4x	72g	556
Weight: 90g		

Fish Finger (grilled)

3g CARBS	40 CALS

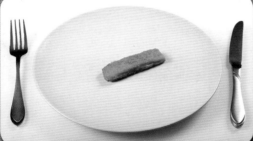

	CARBS	CALS
2x	6g	80
3x	9g	120
4x	12g	160
Weight: 20g		

Fish Goujon (baked)

4g CARBS	56 CALS

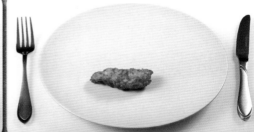

	CARBS	CALS
2x	8g	112
3x	12g	168
4x	16g	224
Weight: 30g		

Scampi (fried)

14g CARBS | **166 CALS**

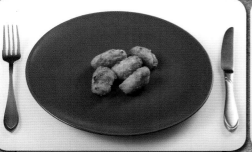

Weight: 70g

Haggis

20g CARBS | **326 CALS**

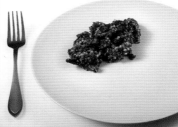

Weight: 105g

29g CARBS | **332 CALS**

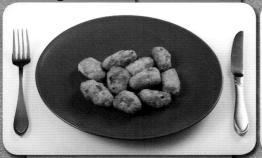

Weight: 140g

40g CARBS | **651 CALS**

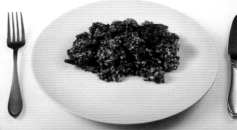

Weight: 210g

43g CARBS | **493 CALS**

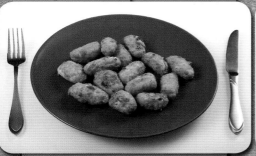

Weight: 208g

60g CARBS | **977 CALS**

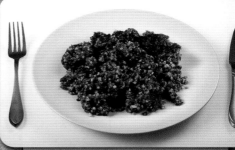

Weight: 315g

Black Pudding (fried)

11g CARBS   **146 CALS**

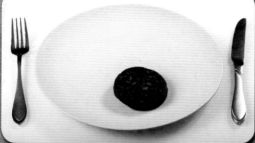

	CARBS	CALS
2x	22g	292
3x	33g	438
4x	44g	584
Weight: 58g		

Chicken Goujon (baked)

6g CARBS   **83 CALS**

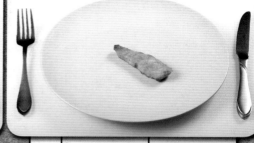

	CARBS	CALS
2x	12g	166
3x	18g	249
4x	24g	332
Weight: 30g		

Sausage (grilled)

2g CARBS   **59 CALS**

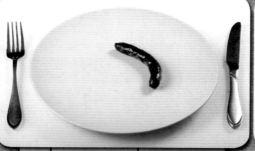

	CARBS	CALS
2x	4g	118
3x	6g	177
4x	8g	236
Weight: 20g (thin)		

5g CARBS   **162 CALS**

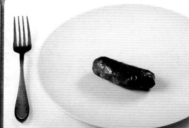

	CARBS	CALS
2x	10g	324
3x	15g	486
4x	20g	648
Weight: 55g (thick)		

Chicken Kiev (baked)

15g CARBS   **348 CALS**

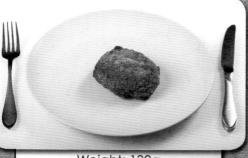

Weight: 130g

30g CARBS   **697 CALS**

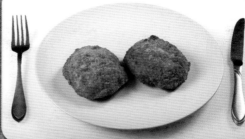

Weight: 260g

Pork Pie

28g CARBS   **432 CALS**

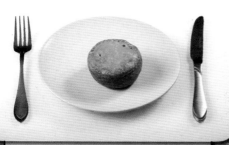

Weight: 119g

76g CARBS   **1162 CALS**

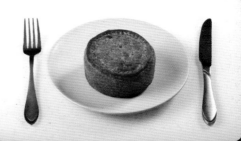

Weight: 320g

Scotch Egg

8g CARBS   **145 CALS**

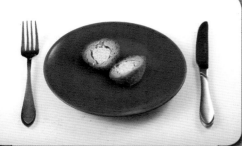

Weight: 60g

16g CARBS   **289 CALS**

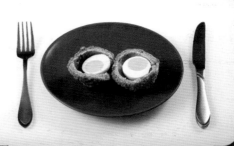

Weight: 120g

Cornish Pasty

8g CARBS   **83 CALS**

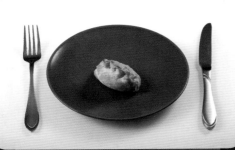

Weight: 31g

41g CARBS   **433 CALS**

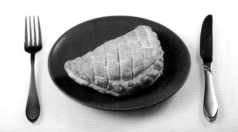

Weight: 162g

49g CARBS   **518 CALS**

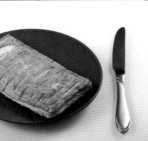

Weight: 194g

109g CARBS   **1159 CALS**

Weight: 434g

Sausage Roll

16g CARBS   **241 CALS**

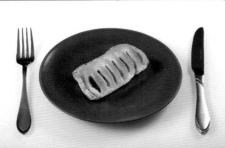

Weight: 63g

31g CARBS   **475 CALS**

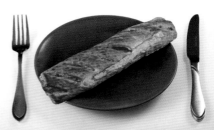

Weight: 124g

Sausages & Beans (tinned)

10g CARBS   **76 CALS**

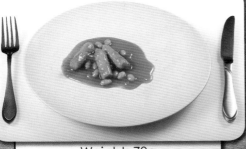

Weight: 70g

20g CARBS   **152 CALS**

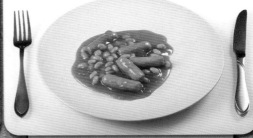

Weight: 140g

30g CARBS   **228 CALS**

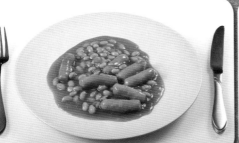

Weight: 210g (half tin)

40g CARBS   **310 CALS**

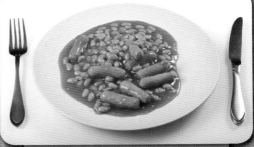

Weight: 285g

50g CARBS   **386 CALS**

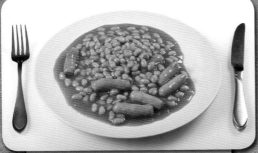

Weight: 355g

60g CARBS   **462 CALS**

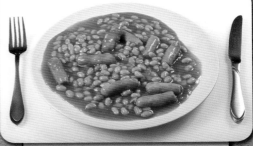

Weight: 425g (full tin)

Cassava Chips (deep fried)

23g CARBS | **122 CALS**

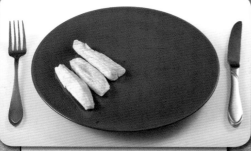

Weight: 45g

47g CARBS | **246 CALS**

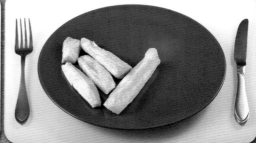

Weight: 91g

71g CARBS | **367 CALS**

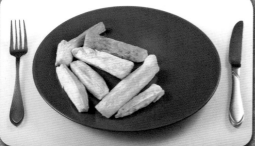

Weight: 136g

95g CARBS | **491 CALS**

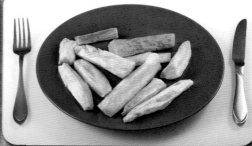

Weight: 182g

119g CARBS | **616 CALS**

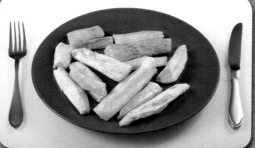

Weight: 228g

141g CARBS | **734 CALS**

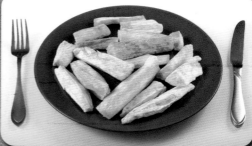

Weight: 272g

Chips (deep fried)

12g CARBS   **90 CALS**

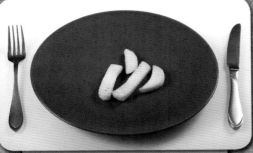

Weight: 33g

36g CARBS   **270 CALS**

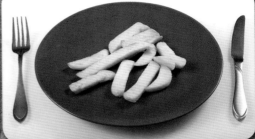

Weight: 99g

59g CARBS   **450 CALS**

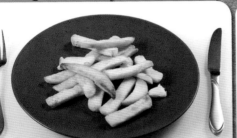

Weight: 165g

83g CARBS   **628 CALS**

Weight: 230g

106g CARBS   **805 CALS**

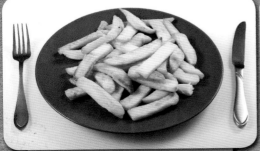

Weight: 295g

130g CARBS   **983 CALS**

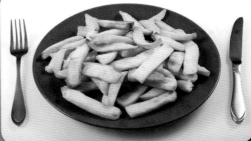

Weight: 360g

Chips (oven)

10g CARBS   **53 CALS**

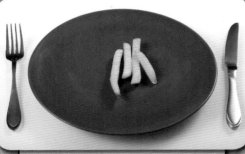

Weight: 33g

30g CARBS   **162 CALS**

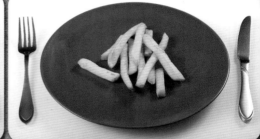

Weight: 100g

50g CARBS   **272 CALS**

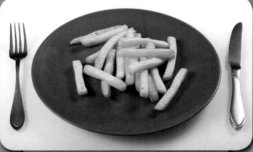

Weight: 168g

70g CARBS   **381 CALS**

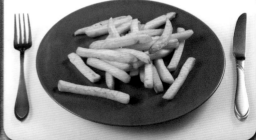

Weight: 235g

90g CARBS   **491 CALS**

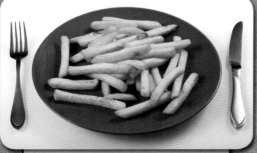

Weight: 303g

110g CARBS   **599 CALS**

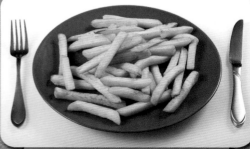

Weight: 370g

Dauphinoise Potatoes

10g CARBS | **178 CALS**

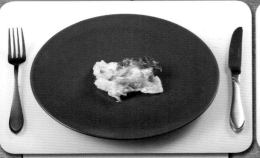

Weight: 72g

20g CARBS | **363 CALS**

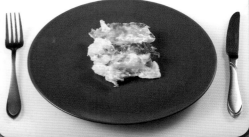

Weight: 147g

30g CARBS | **548 CALS**

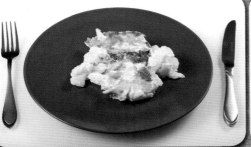

Weight: 222g

40g CARBS | **734 CALS**

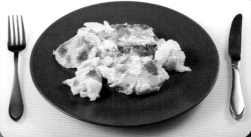

Weight: 297g

50g CARBS | **921 CALS**

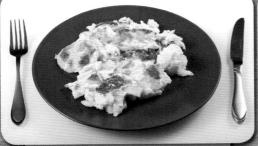

Weight: 373g

60g CARBS | **1107 CALS**

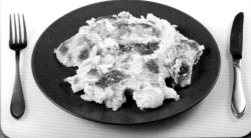

Weight: 448g

Gnocchi

27g CARBS | **122 CALS**

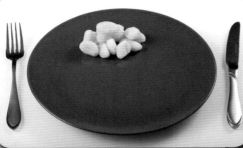

Weight: 80g

55g CARBS | **245 CALS**

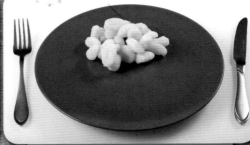

Weight: 160g

82g CARBS | **367 CALS**

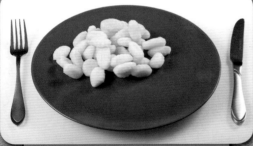

Weight: 240g

110g CARBS | **493 CALS**

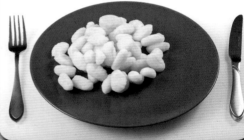

Weight: 322g

137g CARBS | **615 CALS**

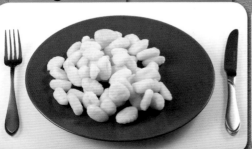

Weight: 402g

164g CARBS | **737 CALS**

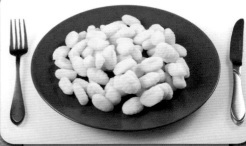

Weight: 482g

Jacket Potato (baked with skin)

20g CARBS | **90 CALS**

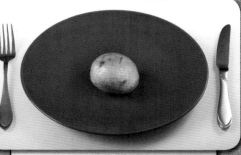

Weight: 95g

35g CARBS | **152 CALS**

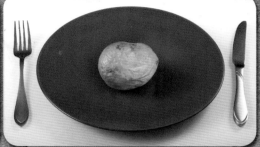

Weight: 158g

45g CARBS | **200 CALS**

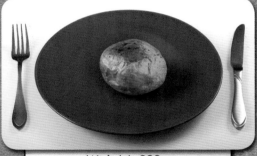

Weight: 220g

60g CARBS | **266 CALS**

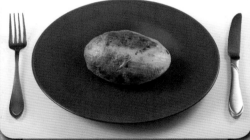

Weight: 284g

75g CARBS | **333 CALS**

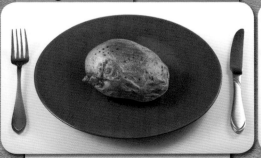

Weight: 348g

90g CARBS | **386 CALS**

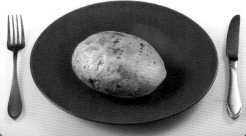

Weight: 410g

Mashed Potato (with butter)

19g CARBS   **125 CALS**

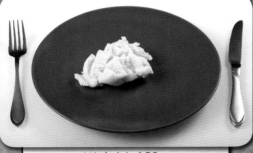

Weight: 120g

36g CARBS   **244 CALS**

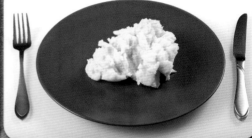

Weight: 235g

55g CARBS   **369 CALS**

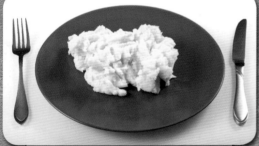

Weight: 355g

73g CARBS   **489 CALS**

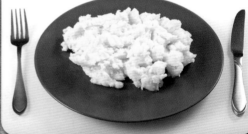

Weight: 470g

91g CARBS   **614 CALS**

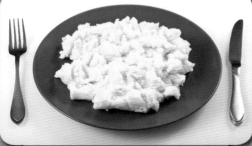

Weight: 590g

109g CARBS   **733 CALS**

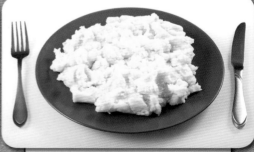

Weight: 705g

New Potatoes (boiled)

10g CARBS   **43 CALS**

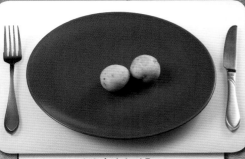

Weight: 65g

20g CARBS   **86 CALS**

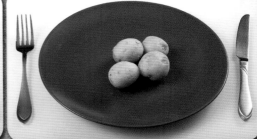

Weight: 130g

30g CARBS   **129 CALS**

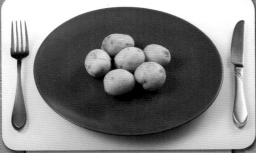

Weight: 195g

40g CARBS   **172 CALS**

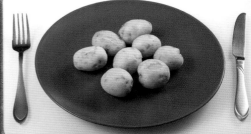

Weight: 260g

60g CARBS   **257 CALS**

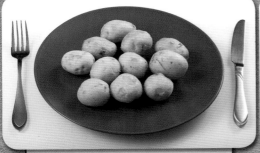

Weight: 390g

80g CARBS   **343 CALS**

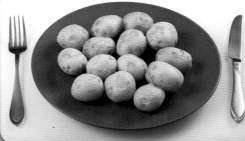

Weight: 520g

Potato Faces (baked)

10g CARBS   **72 CALS**

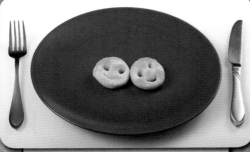

Weight: 34g

21g CARBS   **145 CALS**

Weight: 68g

31g CARBS   **217 CALS**

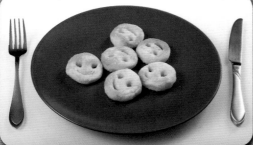

Weight: 102g

42g CARBS   **290 CALS**

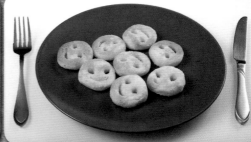

Weight: 136g

52g CARBS   **362 CALS**

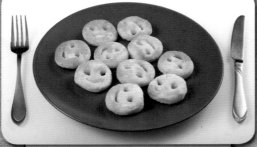

Weight: 170g

63g CARBS   **435 CALS**

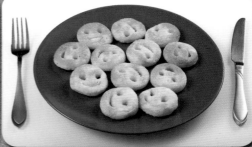

Weight: 204g

Roast Potatoes

10g CARBS | **57** CALS

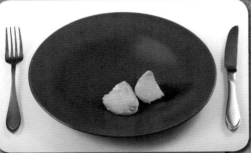

Weight: 38g

25g CARBS | **142** CALS

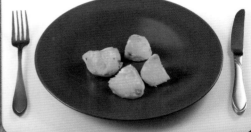

Weight: 95g

40g CARBS | **231** CALS

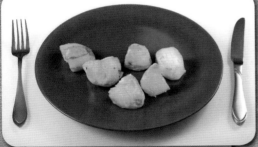

Weight: 155g

55g CARBS | **316** CALS

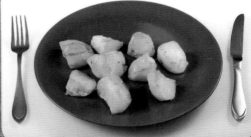

Weight: 212g

70g CARBS | **402** CALS

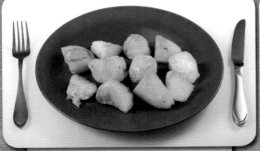

Weight: 270g

85g CARBS | **492** CALS

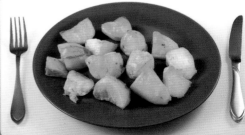

Weight: 330g

Sauté Potatoes (baked)

10g CARBS   **56 CALS**

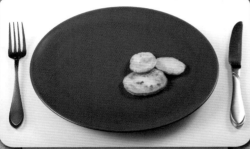

Weight: 28g

20g CARBS   **109 CALS**

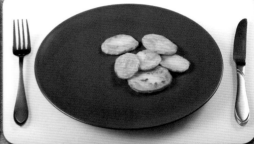

Weight: 55g

30g CARBS   **159 CALS**

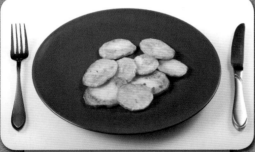

Weight: 80g

40g CARBS   **215 CALS**

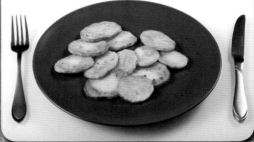

Weight: 108g

50g CARBS   **269 CALS**

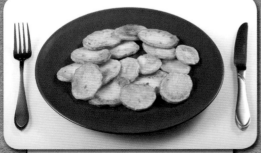

Weight: 135g

60g CARBS   **322 CALS**

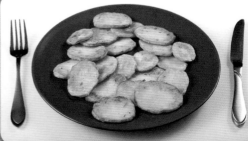

Weight: 162g

Sweet Potatoes (baked)

15g CARBS | **63 CALS**

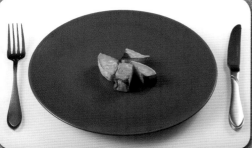

Weight: 55g

30g CARBS | **124 CALS**

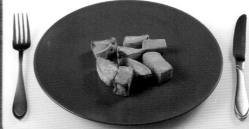

Weight: 108g

45g CARBS | **184 CALS**

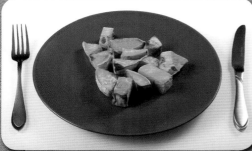

Weight: 160g

60g CARBS | **247 CALS**

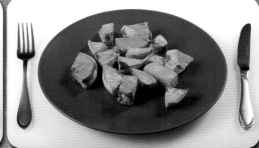

Weight: 215g

75g CARBS | **311 CALS**

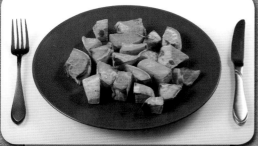

Weight: 270g

90g CARBS | **370 CALS**

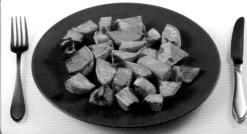

Weight: 322g

Wedges (baked)

13g CARBS   **78 CALS**

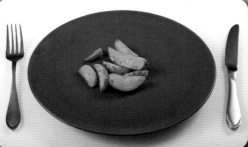

Weight: 55g

25g CARBS   **156 CALS**

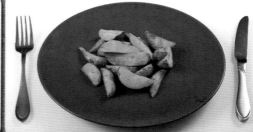

Weight: 110g

38g CARBS   **234 CALS**

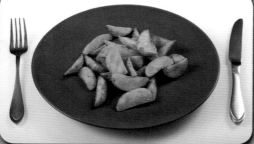

Weight: 165g

51g CARBS   **312 CALS**

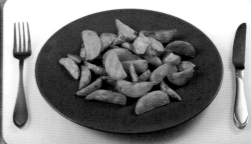

Weight: 220g

62g CARBS   **383 CALS**

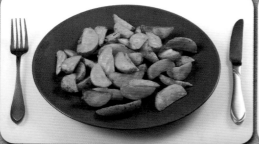

Weight: 270g

75g CARBS   **462 CALS**

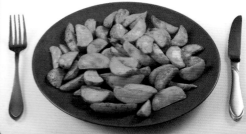

Weight: 325g

Hash Brown (baked)

10g CARBS | **83 CALS**

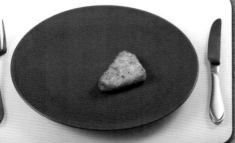

	CARBS	CALS
2x	20g	166
3x	30g	249
4x	40g	332
Weight: 44g		

Potato Croquette (fried)

5g CARBS | **47 CALS**

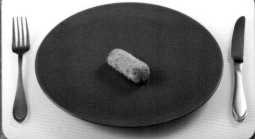

	CARBS	CALS
2x	10g	94
3x	15g	141
4x	20g	188
Weight: 22g		

Potato Rosti (baked)

20g CARBS | **155 CALS**

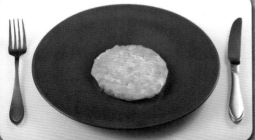

	CARBS	CALS
2x	40g	310
3x	60g	465
4x	80g	620
Weight: 80g		

Potato Waffle (baked)

15g CARBS | **119 CALS**

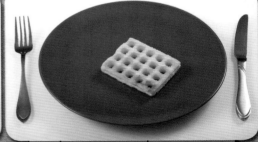

	CARBS	CALS
2x	30g	238
3x	45g	357
4x	60g	476
Weight: 49g		

Bulgur Wheat

20g CARBS   **94 CALS**

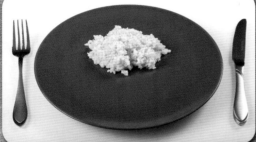

Weight: 100g

40g CARBS   **188 CALS**

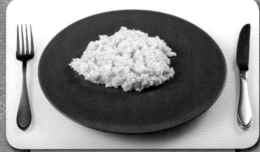

Weight: 200g

60g CARBS   **277 CALS**

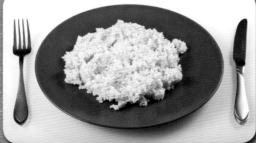

Weight: 295g

Quinoa

20g CARBS   **109 CALS**

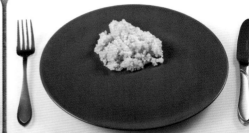

Weight: 85g

40g CARBS   **220 CALS**

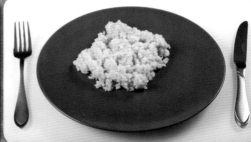

Weight: 172g

60g CARBS   **333 CALS**

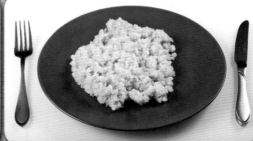

Weight: 260g

Couscous

10g CARBS   **50 CALS**

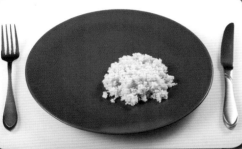

Weight: 45g

25g CARBS   **121 CALS**

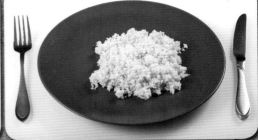

Weight: 110g

40g CARBS   **193 CALS**

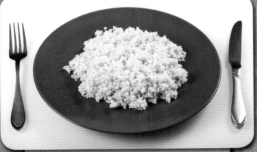

Weight: 175g

55g CARBS   **264 CALS**

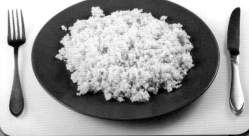

Weight: 240g

70g CARBS   **336 CALS**

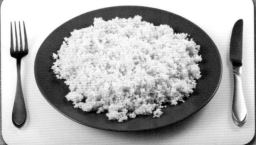

Weight: 305g

85g CARBS   **407 CALS**

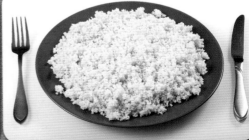

Weight: 370g

Noodles (egg)

20g CARBS   **101 CALS**

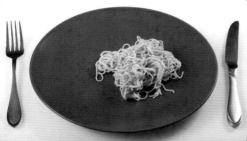

Weight: 58g

40g CARBS   **200 CALS**

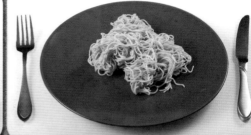

Weight: 115g

60g CARBS   **296 CALS**

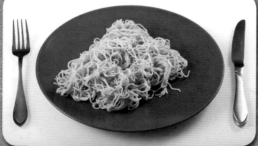

Weight: 170g

80g CARBS   **397 CALS**

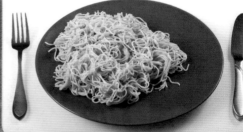

Weight: 228g

100g CARBS   **496 CALS**

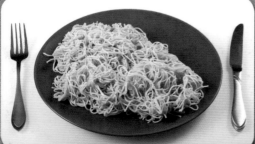

Weight: 285g

120g CARBS   **595 CALS**

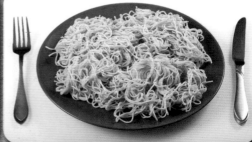

Weight: 342g

Noodles (rice)

20g CARBS · **86 CALS**

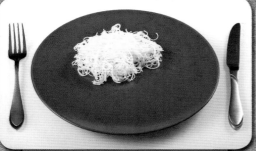

Weight: 70g

40g CARBS · **175 CALS**

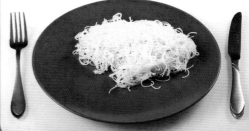

Weight: 142g

60g CARBS · **264 CALS**

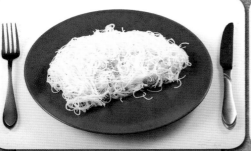

Weight: 215g

80g CARBS · **351 CALS**

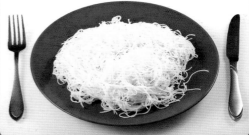

Weight: 285g

100g CARBS · **440 CALS**

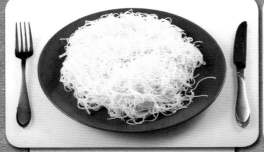

Weight: 358g

120g CARBS · **529 CALS**

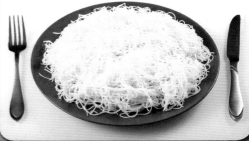

Weight: 430g

Pasta (bows)

10g CARBS   **50 CALS**

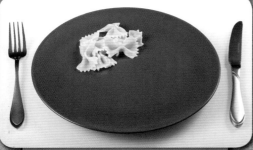

Weight: 30g

30g CARBS   **148 CALS**

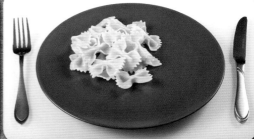

Weight: 88g

50g CARBS   **249 CALS**

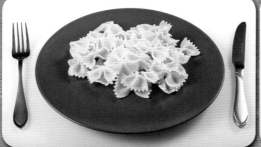

Weight: 148g

70g CARBS   **344 CALS**

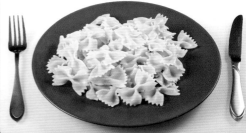

Weight: 205g

90g CARBS   **445 CALS**

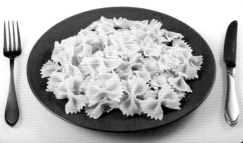

Weight: 265g

110g CARBS   **543 CALS**

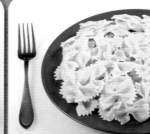

Weight: 323g

Pasta (macaroni)

10g CARBS | 49 CALS
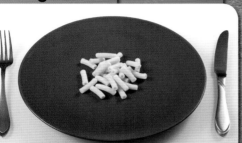
Weight: 32g

30g CARBS | 152 CALS
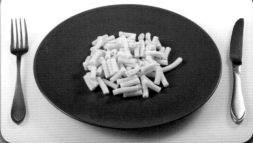
Weight: 100g

50g CARBS | 252 CALS
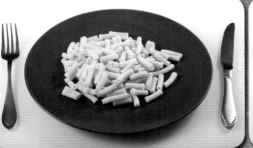
Weight: 166g

70g CARBS | 354 CALS
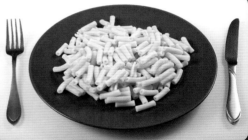
Weight: 233g

90g CARBS | 456 CALS
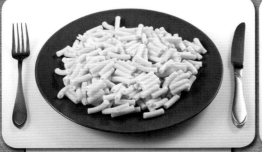
Weight: 300g

110g CARBS | 556 CALS
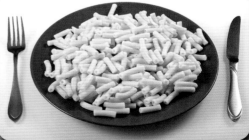
Weight: 366g

Pasta (penne)

10g CARBS   **50 CALS**

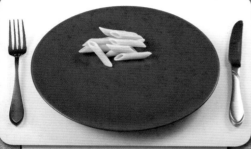

Weight: 30g

30g CARBS   **150 CALS**

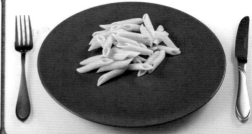

Weight: 90g

50g CARBS   **247 CALS**

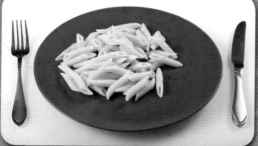

Weight: 148g

70g CARBS   **347 CALS**

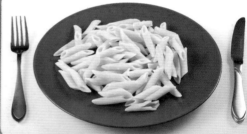

Weight: 208g

90g CARBS   **443 CALS**

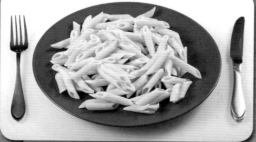

Weight: 265g

110g CARBS   **543 CALS**

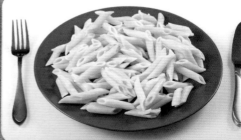

Weight: 325g

Pasta (shells)

10g CARBS **50 CALS**

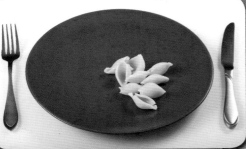

Weight: 30g

30g CARBS **147 CALS**

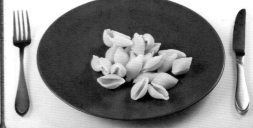

Weight: 88g

50g CARBS **247 CALS**

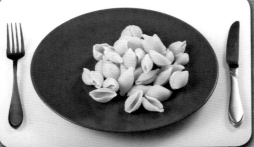

Weight: 148g

70g CARBS **342 CALS**

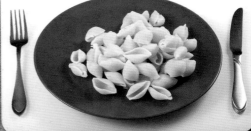

Weight: 205g

90g CARBS **443 CALS**

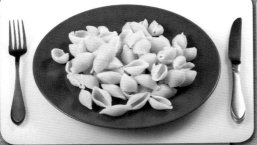

Weight: 265g

110g CARBS **539 CALS**

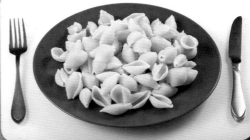

Weight: 323g

Pasta (tagliatelle)

10g CARBS   **53 CALS**

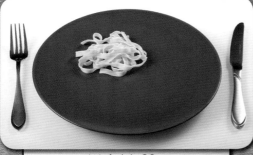

Weight: 30g

30g CARBS   **158 CALS**

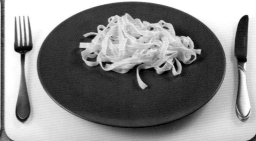

Weight: 90g

50g CARBS   **263 CALS**

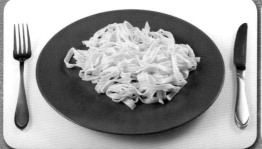

Weight: 150g

70g CARBS   **368 CALS**

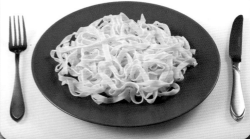

Weight: 210g

90g CARBS   **473 CALS**

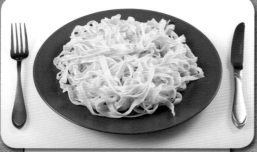

Weight: 270g

110g CARBS   **578 CALS**

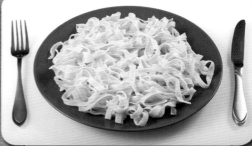

Weight: 330g

Pasta (twirls)

10g CARBS   **50 CALS**

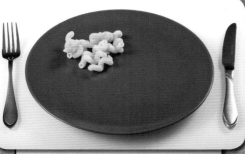

Weight: 30g

30g CARBS   **148 CALS**

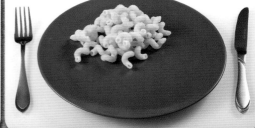

Weight: 88g

50g CARBS   **249 CALS**

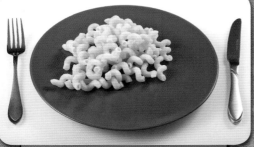

Weight: 148g

70g CARBS   **344 CALS**

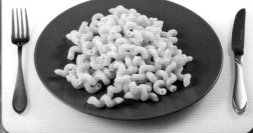

Weight: 205g

90g CARBS   **445 CALS**

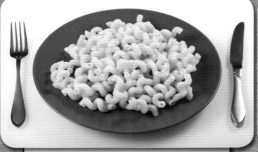

Weight: 265g

110g CARBS   **543 CALS**

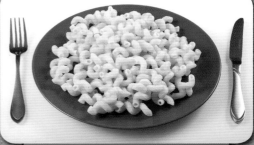

Weight: 323g

Pasta (twists)

10g CARBS | **51 CALS**

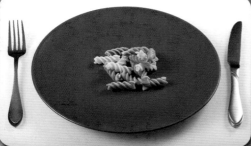

Weight: 30g

30g CARBS | **149 CALS**

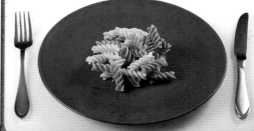

Weight: 88g

50g CARBS | **245 CALS**

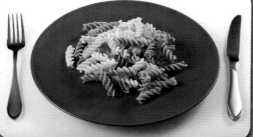

Weight: 145g

70g CARBS | **343 CALS**

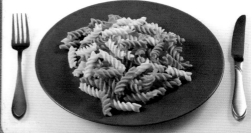

Weight: 203g

90g CARBS | **439 CALS**

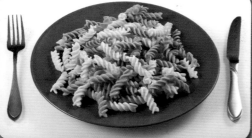

Weight: 260g

110g CARBS | **537 CALS**

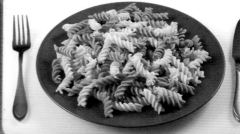

Weight: 318g

Pasta (vermicelli)

10g CARBS   **52 CALS**

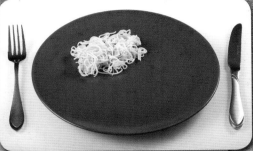

Weight: 40g

30g CARBS   **161 CALS**

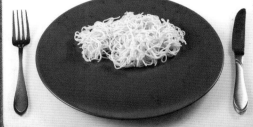

Weight: 125g

50g CARBS   **271 CALS**

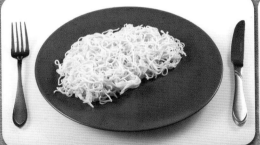

Weight: 210g

70g CARBS   **374 CALS**

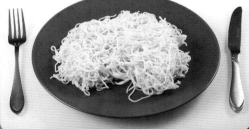

Weight: 290g

90g CARBS   **484 CALS**

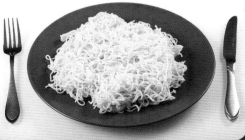

Weight: 375g

110g CARBS   **593 CALS**

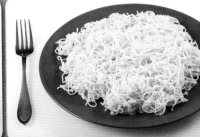

Weight: 460g

Rice (white)

10g CARBS   **44 CALS**

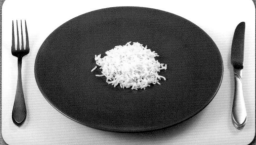

Weight: 32g

30g CARBS   **132 CALS**

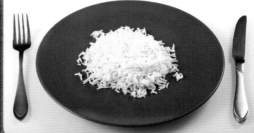

Weight: 96g

50g CARBS   **225 CALS**

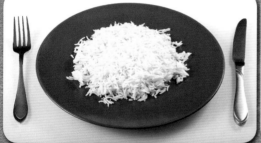

Weight: 163g

70g CARBS   **311 CALS**

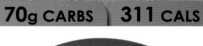
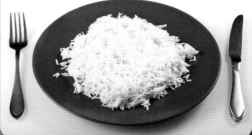

Weight: 225g

90g CARBS   **400 CALS**

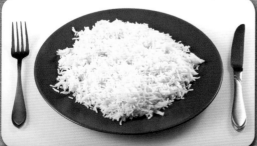

Weight: 290g

110g CARBS   **490 CALS**

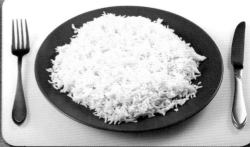

Weight: 355g

Rice (brown)

10g CARBS | **42 CALS**

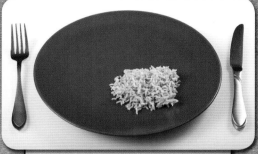

Weight: 30g

30g CARBS | **134 CALS**

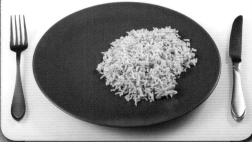

Weight: 95g

50g CARBS | **219 CALS**

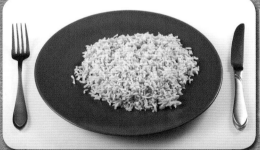

Weight: 155g

70g CARBS | **307 CALS**

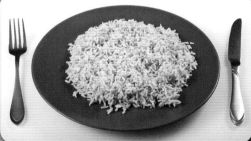

Weight: 218g

90g CARBS | **395 CALS**

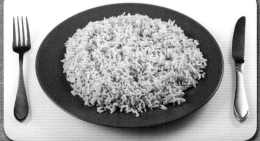

Weight: 280g

110g CARBS | **484 CALS**

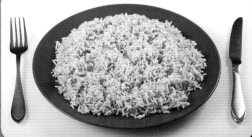

Weight: 343g

Rice (sticky white)

Polenta

21g CARBS **110 CALS**

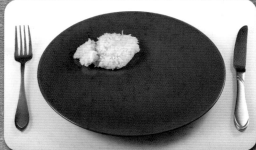

Weight: 80g

10g CARBS **47 CALS**

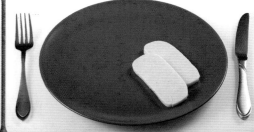

Weight: 65g

41g CARBS **212 CALS**

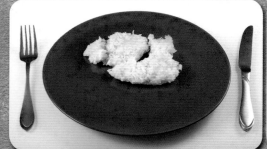

Weight: 155g

20g CARBS **93 CALS**

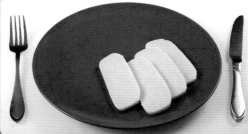

Weight: 130g

63g CARBS **322 CALS**

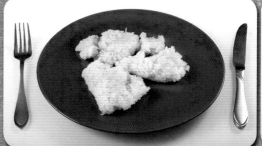

Weight: 235g

30g CARBS **137 CALS**

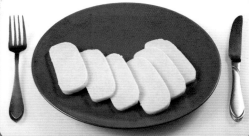

Weight: 190g

Ravioli (fresh, meat-filled)

10g CARBS | **71 CALS**

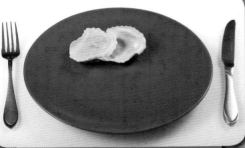

Weight: 40g

30g CARBS | **204 CALS**

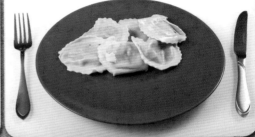

Weight: 115g

50g CARBS | **340 CALS**

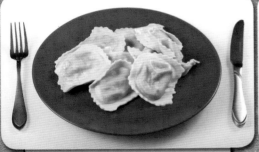

Weight: 192g

70g CARBS | **478 CALS**

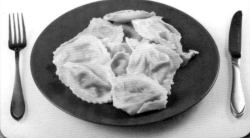

Weight: 270g

90g CARBS | **611 CALS**

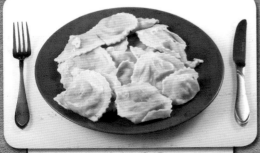

Weight: 345g

110g CARBS | **747 CALS**

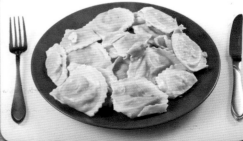

Weight: 422g

Spaghetti (white)

10g CARBS   **52 CALS**

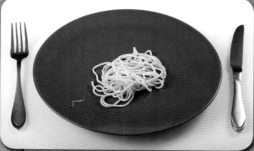

Weight: 33g

30g CARBS   **149 CALS**

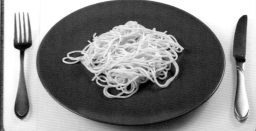

Weight: 95g

50g CARBS   **248 CALS**

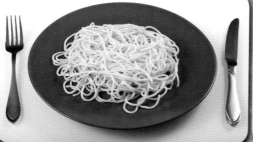

Weight: 158g

70g CARBS   **345 CALS**

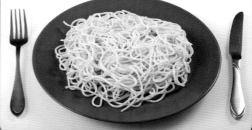

Weight: 220g

90g CARBS   **447 CALS**

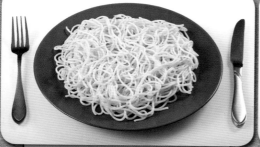

Weight: 285g

110g CARBS   **546 CALS**

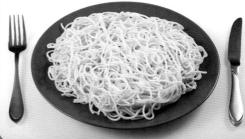

Weight: 348g

Spaghetti (wholemeal)

10g CARBS | **48 CALS**

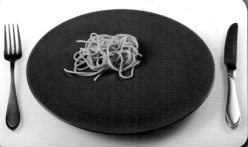

Weight: 33g

30g CARBS | **151 CALS**

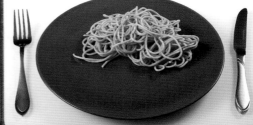

Weight: 105g

50g CARBS | **248 CALS**

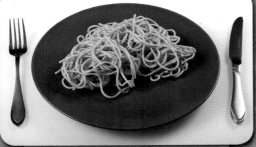

Weight: 172g

70g CARBS | **346 CALS**

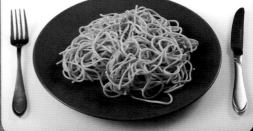

Weight: 240g

90g CARBS | **446 CALS**

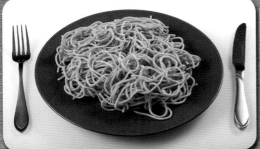

Weight: 310g

110g CARBS | **547 CALS**

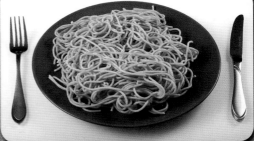

Weight: 380g

Tortellini (fresh, cheese-filled)

13g CARBS   **91 CALS**

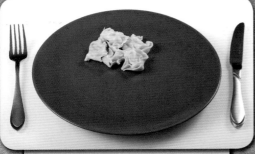

Weight: 42g

45g CARBS   **308 CALS**

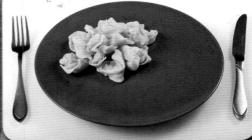

Weight: 142g

76g CARBS   **525 CALS**

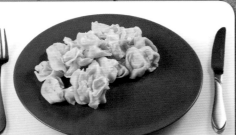

Weight: 242g

107g CARBS   **742 CALS**

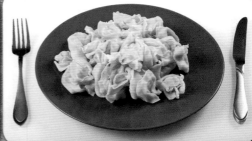

Weight: 342g

139g CARBS   **959 CALS**

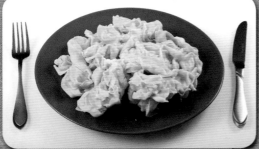

Weight: 442g

170g CARBS   **1176 CALS**

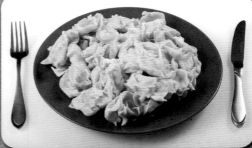

Weight: 542g

Pasta Shapes (tinned)

9g CARBS　**42 CALS**

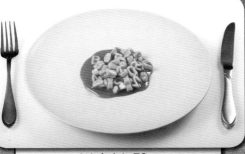

Weight: 70g

17g CARBS　**84 CALS**

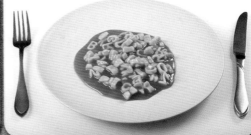

Weight: 140g

26g CARBS　**126 CALS**

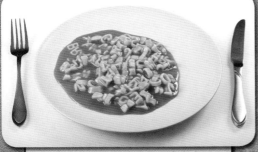

Weight: 210g (half tin)

35g CARBS　**171 CALS**

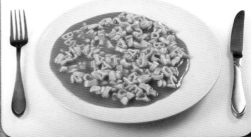

Weight: 285g

44g CARBS　**213 CALS**

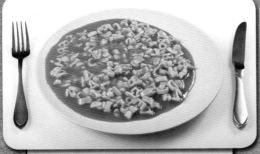

Weight: 355g

52g CARBS　**255 CALS**

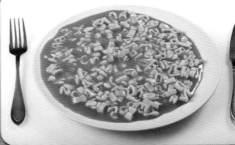

Weight: 425g (full tin)

Ravioli in Tomato Sauce (tinned)

7g CARBS   **49 CALS**

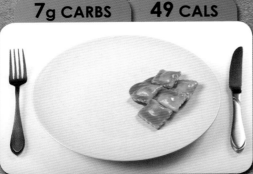

Weight: 70g

14g CARBS   **98 CALS**

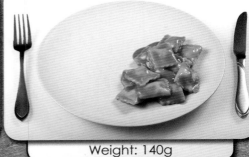

Weight: 140g

22g CARBS   **147 CALS**

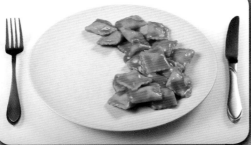

Weight: 210g (half tin)

29g CARBS   **200 CALS**

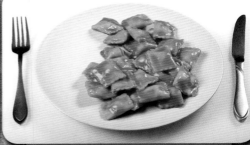

Weight: 285g

37g CARBS   **249 CALS**

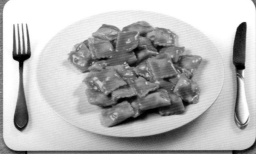

Weight: 355g

44g CARBS   **298 CALS**

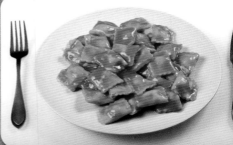

Weight: 425g (full tin)

Spaghetti in Tomato Sauce (tinned)

10g CARBS **45 CALS**

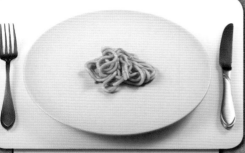

Weight: 70g

20g CARBS **90 CALS**

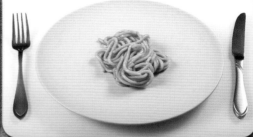

Weight: 140g

30g CARBS **134 CALS**

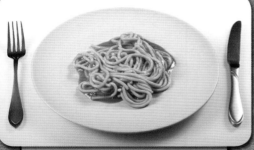

Weight: 210g (half tin)

40g CARBS **182 CALS**

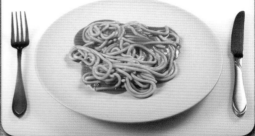

Weight: 285g

50g CARBS **227 CALS**

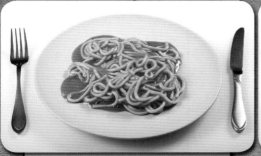

Weight: 355g

60g CARBS **272 CALS**

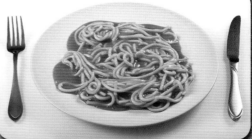

Weight: 425g (full tin)

Spaghetti Hoops in Tomato Sauce (tinned)

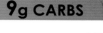

9g CARBS   **41** CALS

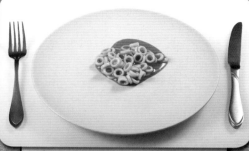

Weight: 70g

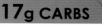

17g CARBS   **82** CALS

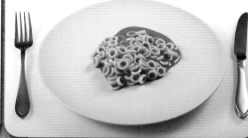

Weight: 140g

26g CARBS   **123** CALS

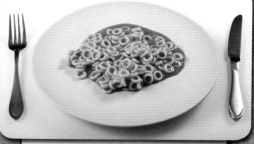

Weight: 210g (half tin)

35g CARBS   **163** CALS

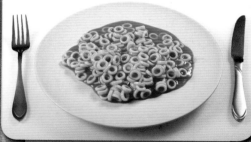

Weight: 280g

43g CARBS   **204** CALS

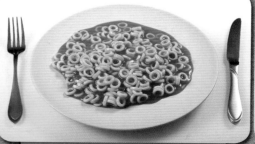

Weight: 350g

52g CARBS   **245** CALS

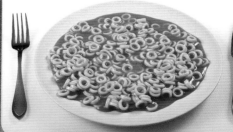

Weight: 420g (full tin)

Crisps

10g CARBS | **95 CALS**

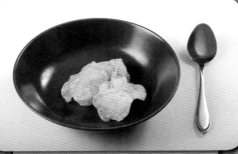

Weight: 18g

20g CARBS | **201 CALS**

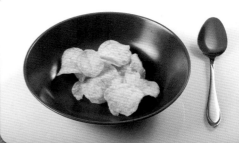

Weight: 38g

30g CARBS | **297 CALS**

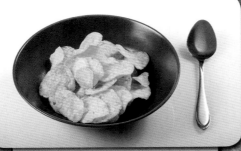

Weight: 56g

40g CARBS | **398 CALS**

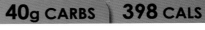
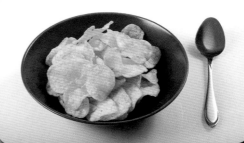

Weight: 75g

50g CARBS | **498 CALS**

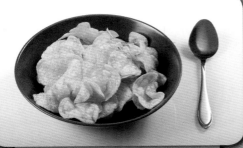

Weight: 94g

60g CARBS | **594 CALS**

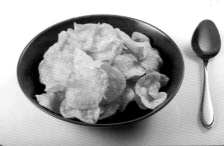

Weight: 112g

Bombay Mix

10g CARBS   **141 CALS**

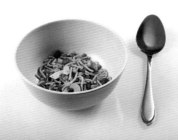

Weight: 28g

20g CARBS   **282 CALS**

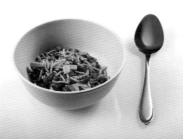

Weight: 56g

30g CARBS   **428 CALS**

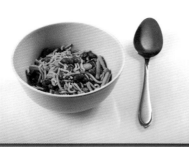

Weight: 85g

Cashew Nuts

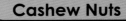

5g CARBS   **171 CALS**

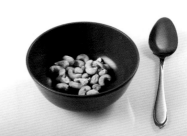

Weight: 28g

10g CARBS   **336 CALS**

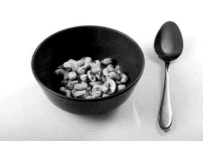

Weight: 55g

15g CARBS   **489 CALS**

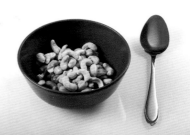

Weight: 80g

Dried Fruit & Nuts

10g CARBS | **99 CALS**

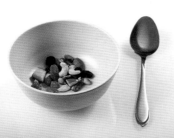

Weight: 22g

20g CARBS | **198 CALS**

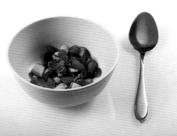

Weight: 44g

30g CARBS | **297 CALS**

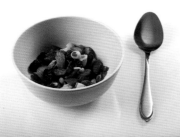

Weight: 66g

Peanuts (roasted)

5g CARBS | **421 CALS**

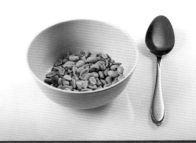

Weight: 70g

10g CARBS | **843 CALS**

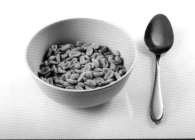

Weight: 140g

15g CARBS | **1264 CALS**

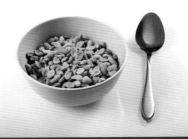

Weight: 210g

Popcorn (with butter)

5g CARBS | **59 CALS**

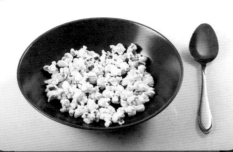

Weight: 10g

10g CARBS | **119 CALS**

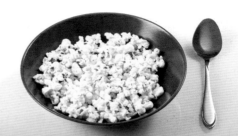

Weight: 20g

15g CARBS | **178 CALS**

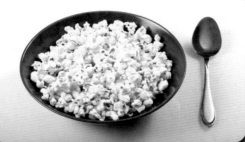

Weight: 30g

20g CARBS | **243 CALS**

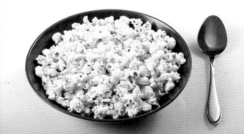

Weight: 41g

25g CARBS | **302 CALS**

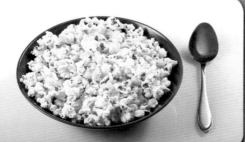

Weight: 51g

30g CARBS | **362 CALS**

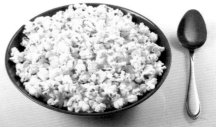

Weight: 61g

Popcorn (sweet)

17g CARBS   **106 CALS**

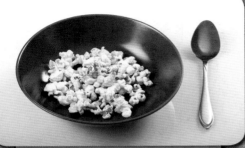

Weight: 22g

35g CARBS   **216 CALS**

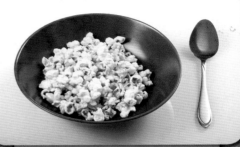

Weight: 45g

53g CARBS   **326 CALS**

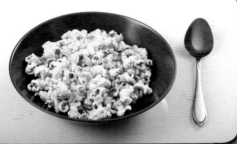

Weight: 68g

70g CARBS   **432 CALS**

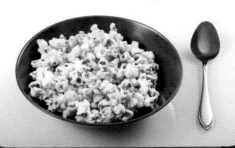

Weight: 90g

88g CARBS   **542 CALS**

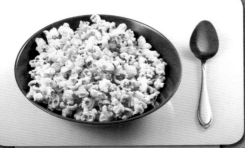

Weight: 113g

105g CARBS   **648 CALS**

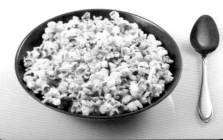

Weight: 135g

Prawn Crackers

5g CARBS | 51 CALS

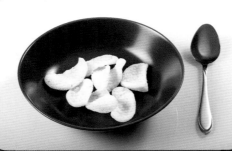

Weight: 9g

10g CARBS | 103 CALS

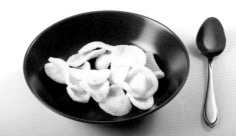

Weight: 18g

20g CARBS | 200 CALS

Weight: 35g

30g CARBS | 296 CALS

Weight: 52g

40g CARBS | 388 CALS

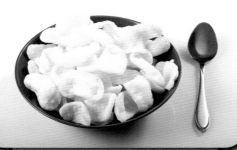

Weight: 68g

50g CARBS | 490 CALS

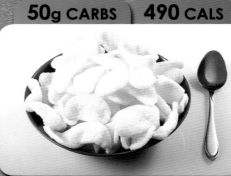

Weight: 86g

Tortilla Chips

10g CARBS   **73 CALS**

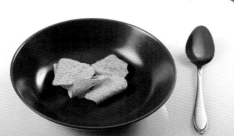

Weight: 16g

30g CARBS   **230 CALS**

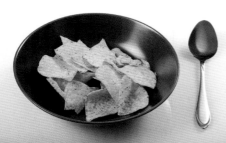

Weight: 50g

60g CARBS   **459 CALS**

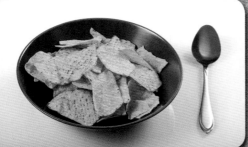

Weight: 100g

Houmous

5g CARBS   **84 CALS**

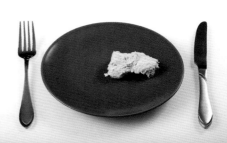

Weight: 45g

10g CARBS   **168 CALS**

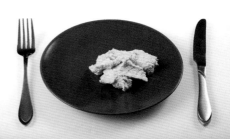

Weight: 90g

15g CARBS   **243 CALS**

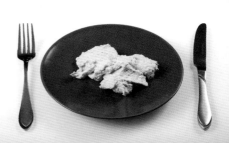

Weight: 130g

Pretzels

10g CARBS   **50 CALS**

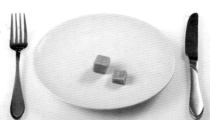

Weight: 13g

21g CARBS   **99 CALS**

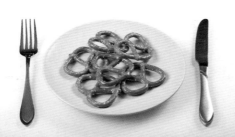

Weight: 26g

32g CARBS   **152 CALS**

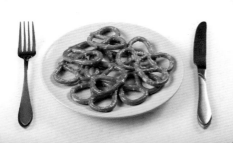

Weight: 40g

Fudge

10g CARBS   **53 CALS**

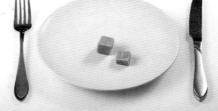

Weight: 12g

20g CARBS   **110 CALS**

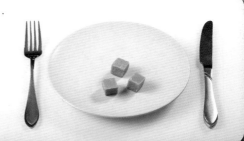

Weight: 25g

30g CARBS   **162 CALS**

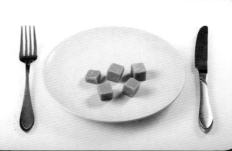

Weight: 37g

Chocolate (milk)

9g CARBS | **83 CALS**

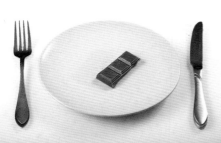

Weight: 16g

19g CARBS | **172 CALS**

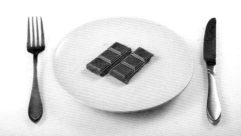

Weight: 33g

28g CARBS | **260 CALS**

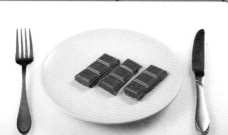

Weight: 50g

38g CARBS | **348 CALS**

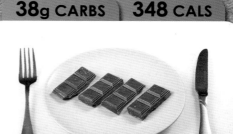

Weight: 67g

48g CARBS | **442 CALS**

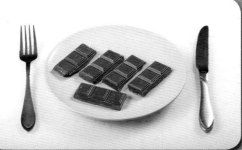

Weight: 85g

57g CARBS | **525 CALS**

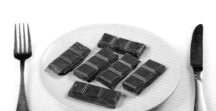

Weight: 101g

Chocolate (dark)

10g CARBS   **82 CALS**

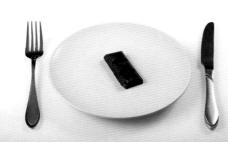

Weight: 16g

20g CARBS   **163 CALS**

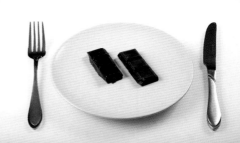

Weight: 32g

30g CARBS   **245 CALS**

Weight: 48g

40g CARBS   **321 CALS**

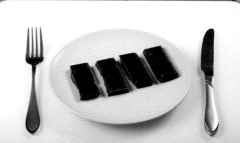

Weight: 63g

50g CARBS   **398 CALS**

Weight: 78g

60g CARBS   **479 CALS**

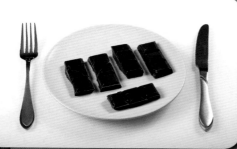

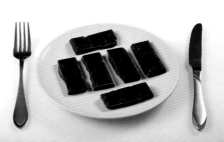

Weight: 94g

Chocolate Mint

9g CARBS   **70 CALS**

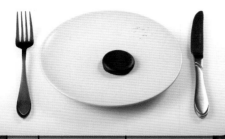

	CARBS	CALS
2x	18g	140
3x	27g	210
4x	36g	280
Weight: 15g		

Licorice Allsorts

9g CARBS   **42 CALS**

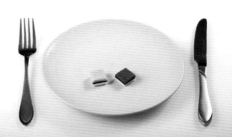

	CARBS	CALS
2x	18g	84
3x	27g	126
4x	36g	168
Weight: 12g		

Individual Chocolate

7g CARBS   **54 CALS**

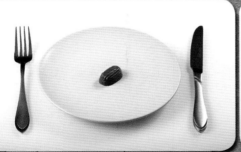

	CARBS	CALS
2x	14g	108
3x	21g	162
4x	28g	216
Weight: 11g		

8g CARBS   **71 CALS**

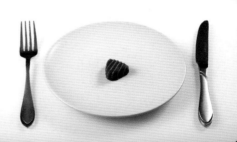

	CARBS	CALS
2x	16g	142
3x	24g	213
4x	32g	284
Weight: 14g		

Cola Bottles

10g CARBS **43 CALS**

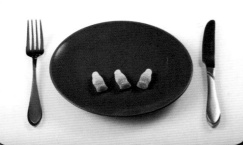

	CARBS	CALS
2x	20g	86
3x	30g	129
4x	40g	172
Weight: 13g		

Jelly Babies

15g CARBS **62 CALS**

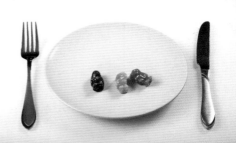

	CARBS	CALS
2x	30g	124
3x	45g	186
4x	60g	248
Weight: 18g		

Jelly Beans

10g CARBS **40 CALS**

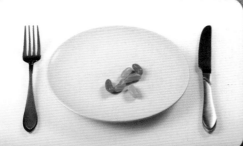

	CARBS	CALS
2x	20g	80
3x	30g	120
4x	40g	160
Weight: 11g		

Wine Gums

10g CARBS **45 CALS**

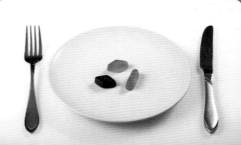

	CARBS	CALS
2x	20g	90
3x	30g	135
4x	40g	180
Weight: 14g		

Fish Stew with Jollof Rice

46g CARBS   **490 CALS**

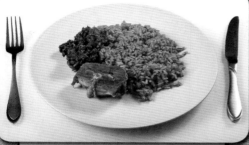

55g fish, 145g rice, 55g veg

96g CARBS   **1024 CALS**

115g fish, 303g rice, 115g veg

142g CARBS   **1513 CALS**

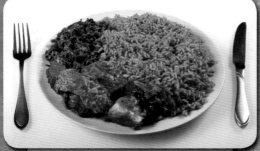

170g fish, 448g rice, 170g veg

Fufu (yam)

49g CARBS   **202 CALS**

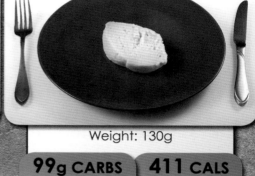

Weight: 130g

99g CARBS   **411 CALS**

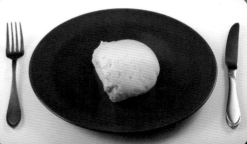

Weight: 265g

140g CARBS   **581 CALS**

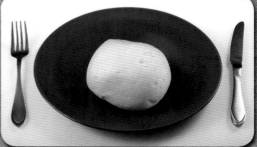

Weight: 375g

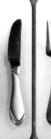

Beef Burger (with cheese)

31g CARBS   **519** CALS

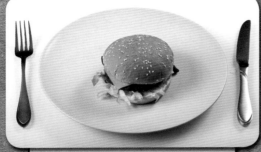

Weight: 181g

French Fries

33g CARBS   **269** CALS

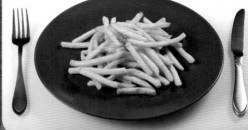

Weight: 96g (small)

Chicken Burger

45g CARBS   **398** CALS

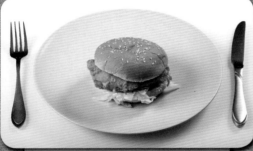

Weight: 168g

54g CARBS   **448** CALS

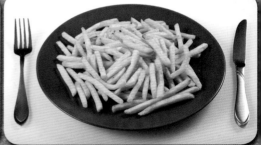

Weight: 160g (medium)

Veggie Burger

41g CARBS   **321** CALS

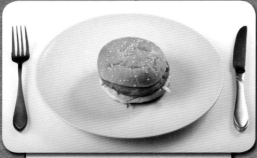

Weight: 158g

77g CARBS   **636** CALS

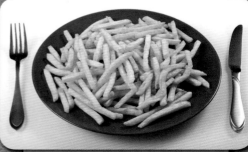

Weight: 227g (large)

* SEE PAGE 14

Caribbean - Fried Fish, Rice & Peas

56g CARBS	555 CALS

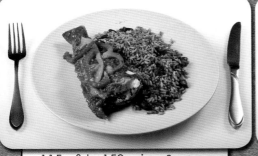

115g fish, 150g rice & peas

113g CARBS	1110 CALS

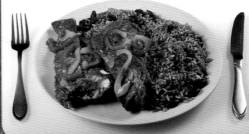

230g fish, 300g rice & peas

Caribbean - Goat & Potato Curry, Rice & Peas

76g CARBS	859 CALS

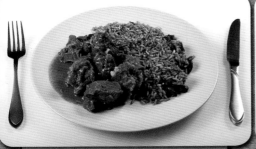

225g curry, 150g rice & peas

154g CARBS	1718 CALS

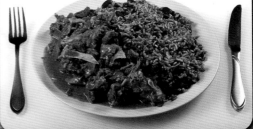

450g curry, 300g rice & peas

Caribbean - Jerk Chicken, Rice & Peas

49g CARBS	511 CALS

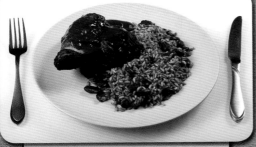

210g chicken, 150g rice & peas

98g CARBS	1023 CALS

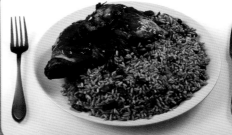

420g chicken, 300g rice & peas

* SEE PAGE 14

Caribbean - Jamaican Beef Patty

| 27g CARBS | 279 CALS | 54g CARBS | 551 CALS |

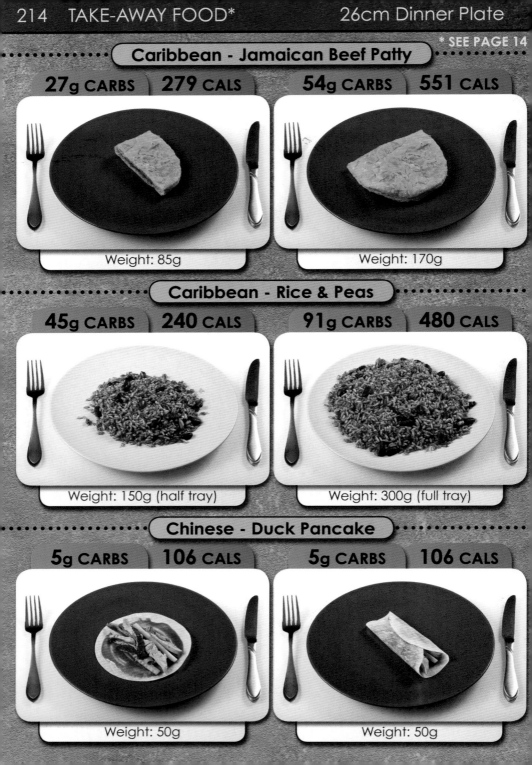

Weight: 85g

Weight: 170g

Caribbean - Rice & Peas

| 45g CARBS | 240 CALS | 91g CARBS | 480 CALS |

Weight: 150g (half tray)

Weight: 300g (full tray)

Chinese - Duck Pancake

| 5g CARBS | 106 CALS | 5g CARBS | 106 CALS |

Weight: 50g

Weight: 50g

* SEE PAGE 14

Chinese - Chicken Balls

5g CARBS   **97 CALS**

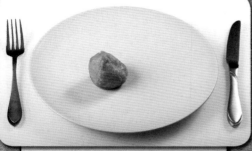

Weight: 38g

20g CARBS   **357 CALS**

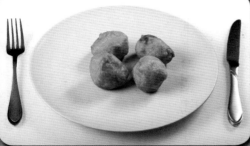

Weight: 140g (half tray)

40g CARBS   **714 CALS**

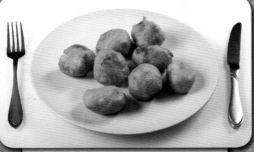

Weight: 280g (full tray)

Chinese - Prawn Toast

5g CARBS   **123 CALS**

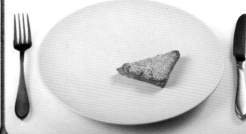

Weight: 32g

10g CARBS   **234 CALS**

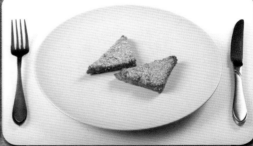

Weight: 61g

15g CARBS   **345 CALS**

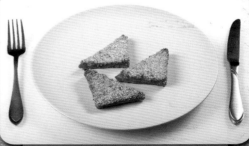

Weight: 90g (full tray)

* SEE PAGE 14

Chinese - Beef Chow Mein

| 40g CARBS | 374 CALS | 80g CARBS | 741 CALS |

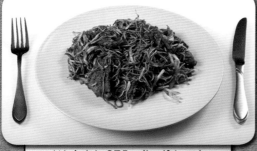
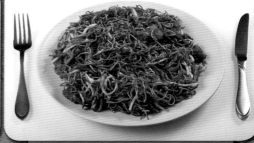

Weight: 275g (half tray)

Weight: 545g (full tray)

Chinese - Chicken Curry

| 5g CARBS | 276 CALS | 10g CARBS | 551 CALS |

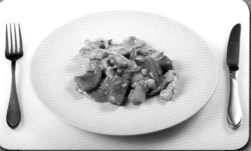
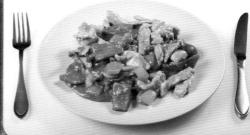

Weight: 190g (half tray)

Weight: 380g (full tray)

Chinese - Singapore Noodles

| 26g CARBS | 223 CALS | 52g CARBS | 447 CALS |

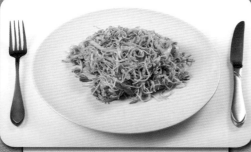
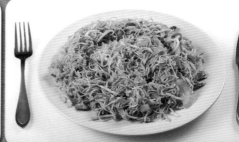

Weight: 205g (half tray)

Weight: 410g (full tray)

* SEE PAGE 14

Chinese - Egg Fried Rice

| 60g CARBS | 335 CALS | 120g CARBS | 670 CALS |

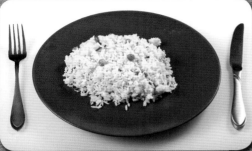
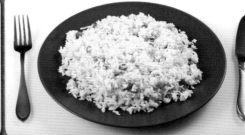

Weight: 180g (half tray)   Weight: 360g (full tray)

Chinese - Spring Roll

| 5g CARBS | 52 CALS | 15g CARBS | 152 CALS |

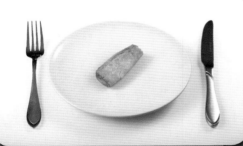
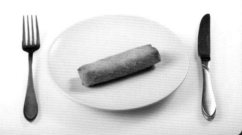

Weight: 24g   Weight: 70g

Chinese - Spare Ribs

| 15g CARBS | 368 CALS | 31g CARBS | 747 CALS |

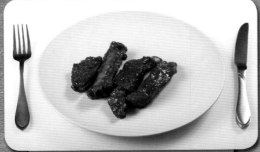
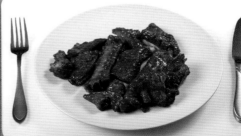

Weight: 150g (half tray)   Weight: 305g (full tray)

* SEE PAGE 14

Chip Shop - Fish

16g CARBS   **333 CALS**

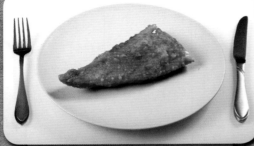

Weight: 135g

39g CARBS   **815 CALS**

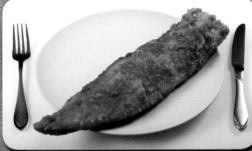

Weight: 330g

Chip Shop - Chips

40g CARBS   **311 CALS**

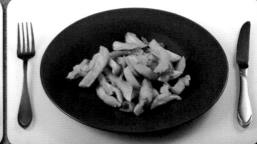

Weight: 130g

80g CARBS   **626 CALS**

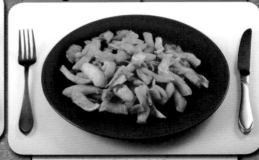

Weight: 262g

Battered Sausage

25g CARBS   **421 CALS**

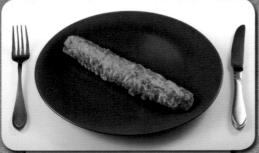

Weight: 137g

120g CARBS   **944 CALS**

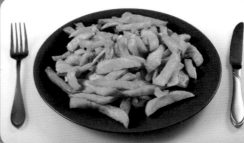

Weight: 395g

* SEE PAGE 14

Indian - Onion Bhaji

15g CARBS | **205 CALS**

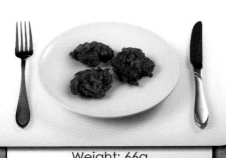

Weight: 66g

15g CARBS | **205 CALS**

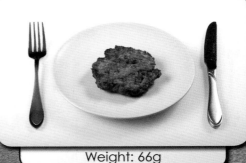

Weight: 66g

Indian - Pakora

5g CARBS | **52 CALS**

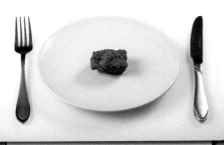

Weight: 22g

10g CARBS | **106 CALS**

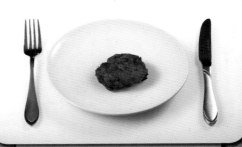

Weight: 45g

Indian - Samosa (meat)

6g CARBS | **82 CALS**

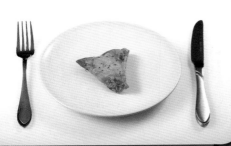

Weight: 30g

11g CARBS | **158 CALS**

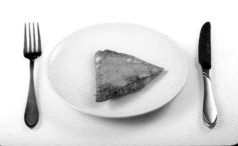

Weight: 58g

* SEE PAGE 14

Indian - Chicken Tikka Masala

5g CARBS | **290 CALS**

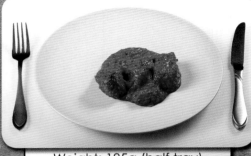

Weight: 185g (half tray)

10g CARBS | **581 CALS**

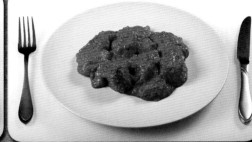

Weight: 370g (full tray)

Indian - King Prawn Bhuna

4g CARBS | **205 CALS**

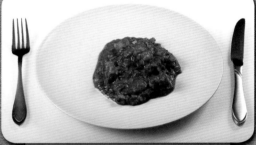

Weight: 175g (half tray)

8g CARBS | **410 CALS**

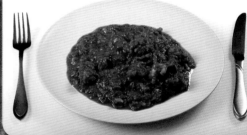

Weight: 350g (full tray)

Indian - Lamb Rogan Josh

7g CARBS | **261 CALS**

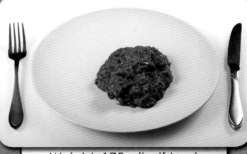

Weight: 175g (half tray)

14g CARBS | **522 CALS**

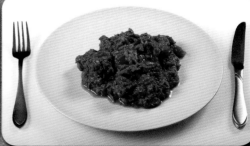

Weight: 350g (full tray)

* SEE PAGE 14

Indian - Bombay Potatoes

21g CARBS | **177 CALS**

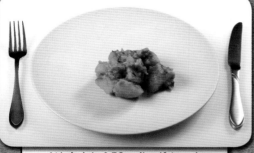

Weight: 150g (half tray)

41g CARBS | **354 CALS**

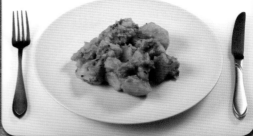

Weight: 300g (full tray)

Indian - Sag Aloo Gobi

9g CARBS | **124 CALS**

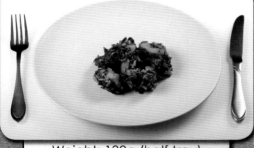

Weight: 130g (half tray)

18g CARBS | **247 CALS**

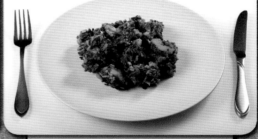

Weight: 260g (full tray)

Indian - Sweet Mango Chutney

8g CARBS | **30 CALS**

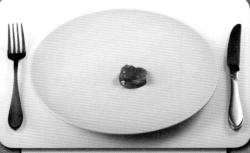

Weight: 16g

16g CARBS | **62 CALS**

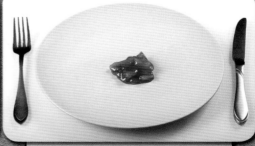

Weight: 33g

Doner Kebab

50g CARBS | **580 CALS**

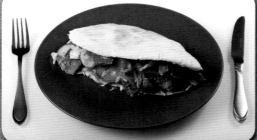

Weight: 250g (small)

80g CARBS | **1053 CALS**

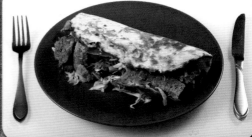

Weight: 415g (large)

Shish Kebab

50g CARBS | **435 CALS**

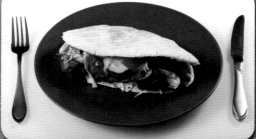

Weight: 250g (small)

80g CARBS | **762 CALS**

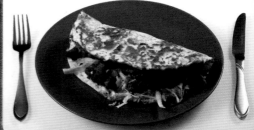

Weight: 415g (large)

Falafel in Pitta

60g CARBS | **372 CALS**

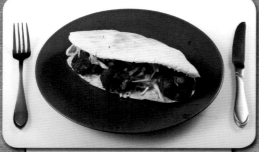

Weight: 200g (small)

100g CARBS | **647 CALS**

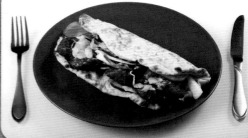

Weight: 350g (large)

Pizza (meat, deep pan)

21g CARBS   176 CALS

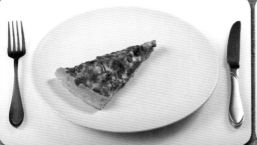

	CARBS	CALS
2x	42g	352
3x	63g	528
4x	84g	704
Weight: 70g		

41g CARBS   353 CALS

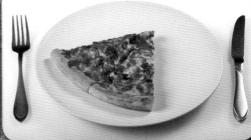

	CARBS	CALS
2x	82g	706
3x	123g	1059
4x	164g	1412
Weight: 140g		

62g CARBS   524 CALS

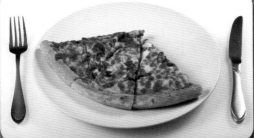

	CARBS	CALS
2x	124g	1048
3x	186g	1572
4x	248g	2096
Weight: 208g		

82g CARBS   698 CALS

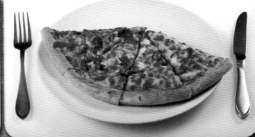

	CARBS	CALS
2x	164g	1396
3x	246g	2094
4x	328g	2792
Weight: 277g		

Pizza (vegetable, thin crust)

13g CARBS · 126 CALS

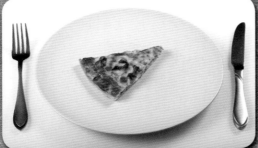

	CARBS	CALS
2x	26g	252
3x	39g	378
4x	52g	504
Weight: 50g		

26g CARBS · 252 CALS

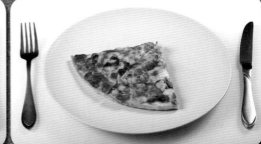

	CARBS	CALS
2x	52g	504
3x	78g	756
4x	104g	1008
Weight: 100g		

39g CARBS · 378 CALS

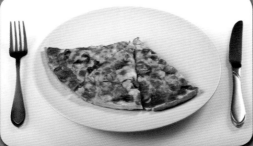

	CARBS	CALS
2x	78	756
3x	117g	1134
4x	156g	1512
Weight: 150g		

52g CARBS · 504 CALS

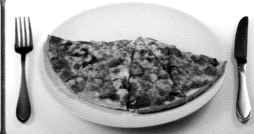

	CARBS	CALS
2x	104g	1008
3x	156g	1512
4x	208g	2016
Weight: 200g		

* SEE PAGE 14

Pizza (pepperoni, stuffed crust)

20g CARBS | **170 CALS**

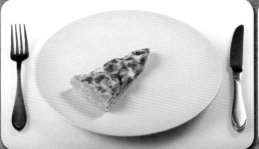

	CARBS	CALS
2x	40g	340
3x	60g	510
4x	80g	680
Weight: 65g		

40g CARBS | **339 CALS**

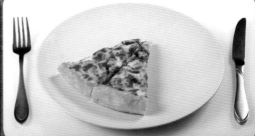

	CARBS	CALS
2x	80g	678
3x	120g	1017
4x	160g	1356
Weight: 130g		

60g CARBS | **517 CALS**

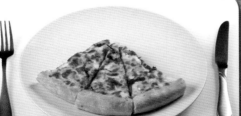

	CARBS	CALS
2x	120g	1034
3x	180g	1551
4x	240g	2068
Weight: 198g		

80g CARBS | **684 CALS**

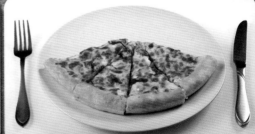

	CARBS	CALS
2x	160g	1368
3x	240g	2052
4x	320g	2736
Weight: 262g		

* SEE PAGE 14

Thai - Green Curry

7g CARBS | **271 CALS**

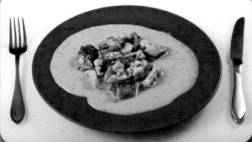

Weight: 195g (half tray)

13g CARBS | **542 CALS**

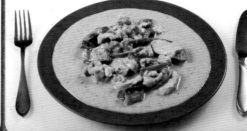

Weight: 390g (full tray)

Thai - Phad Thai

49g CARBS | **325 CALS**

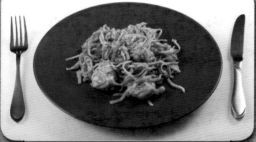

Weight: 200g (half tray)

97g CARBS | **649 CALS**

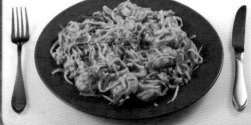

Weight: 400g (full tray)

Thai - Pineapple, Chicken & Prawn Rice

69g CARBS | **483 CALS**

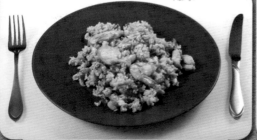

Weight: 250g (half tray)

139g CARBS | **965 CALS**

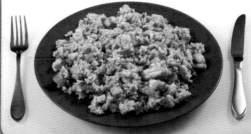

Weight: 500g (full tray)

* SEE PAGE 10

Baked Beans *

10g CARBS | **55 CALS**

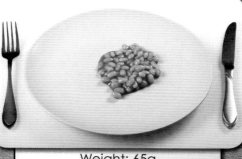

Weight: 65g

20g CARBS | **109 CALS**

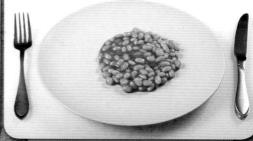

Weight: 130g

30g CARBS | **164 CALS**

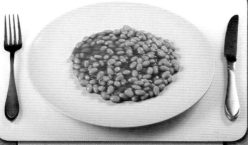

Weight: 195g (half tin)

40g CARBS | **218 CALS**

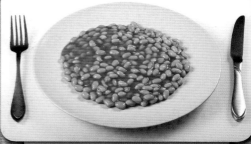

Weight: 260g

50g CARBS | **273 CALS**

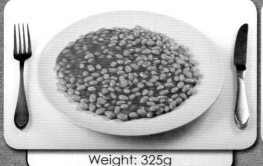

Weight: 325g

60g CARBS | **328 CALS**

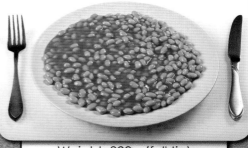

Weight: 390g (full tin)

* SEE PAGE 10

Chick Peas *

5g CARBS   35 CALS

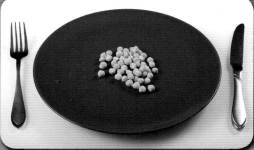

Weight: 30g

10g CARBS   69 CALS

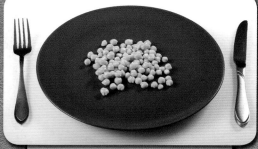

Weight: 60g

20g CARBS   144 CALS

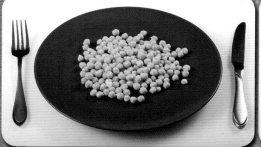

Weight: 125g

Lentils *

10g CARBS   63 CALS

Weight: 60g

20g CARBS   126 CALS

Weight: 120g

30g CARBS   189 CALS

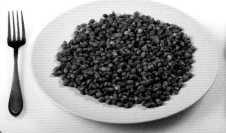

Weight: 180g

* SEE PAGE 10

Kidney Beans *

5g CARBS	30 CALS

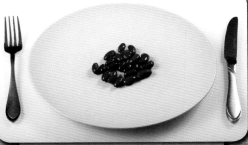

Weight: 30g

10g CARBS	55 CALS

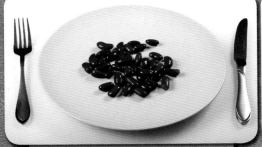

Weight: 55g

20g CARBS	115 CALS

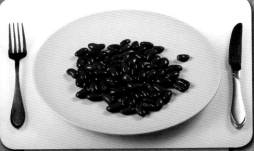

Weight: 115g

Mung Beans *

5g CARBS	27 CALS

Weight: 30g

10g CARBS	59 CALS

Weight: 65g

15g CARBS	86 CALS

Weight: 95g

* SEE PAGE 10

 Peas *   **Mushy Peas ***

5g CARBS   **35** CALS   **10**g CARBS   **61** CALS

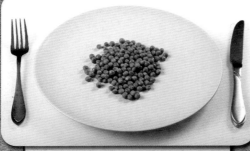   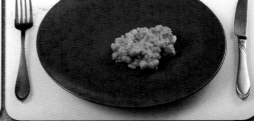

Weight: 50g   Weight: 75g

10g CARBS   **69** CALS   **20**g CARBS   **117** CALS

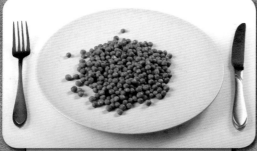   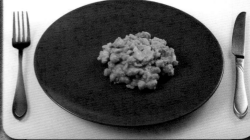

Weight: 100g   Weight: 145g

15g CARBS   **104** CALS   **40**g CARBS   **243** CALS

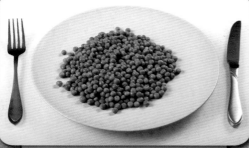   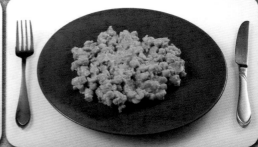

Weight: 150g   Weight: 300g

* SEE PAGE 10

Parsnips (baked) *

13g CARBS | 83 CALS

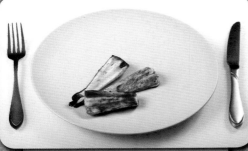

Weight: 60g

24g CARBS | 160 CALS

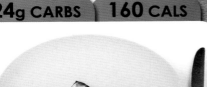

Weight: 115g

37g CARBS | 243 CALS

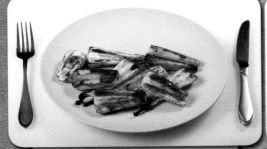

Weight: 175g

Butternut Squash (baked) *

10g CARBS | 42 CALS

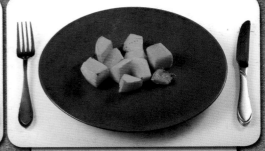

Weight: 130g

20g CARBS | 85 CALS

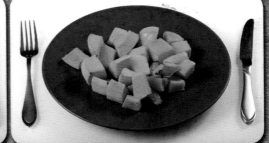

Weight: 265g

30g CARBS | 128 CALS

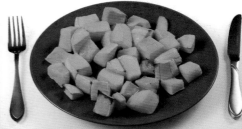

Weight: 400g

* SEE PAGE 10

Sweetcorn *

10g CARBS   **46 CALS**

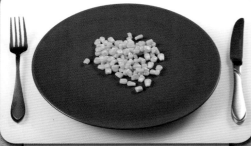

Weight: 38g

20g CARBS   **92 CALS**

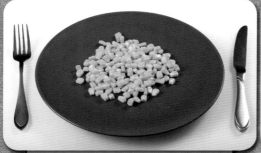

Weight: 75g

40g CARBS   **183 CALS**

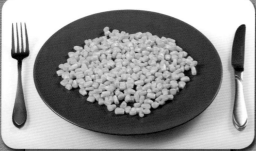

Weight: 150g

Corn on the Cob *

5g CARBS   **29 CALS**

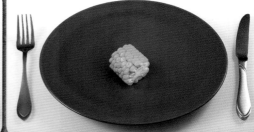

Weight: 44g

10g CARBS   **56 CALS**

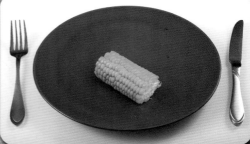

Weight: 85g

20g CARBS   **112 CALS**

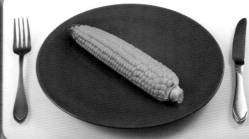

Weight: 170g

Plantain (fried)

20g CARBS | **112** CALS

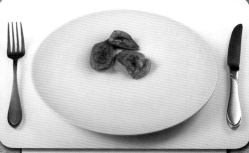

Weight: 42g

40g CARBS | **224** CALS

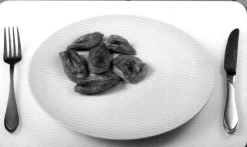

Weight: 84g

60g CARBS | **336** CALS

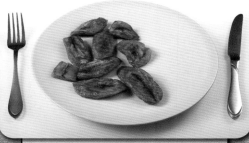

Weight: 126g

Yam (boiled)

20g CARBS | **80** CALS

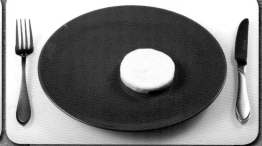

Weight: 60g

40g CARBS | **160** CALS

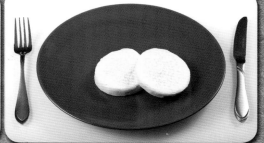

Weight: 120g

60g CARBS | **242** CALS

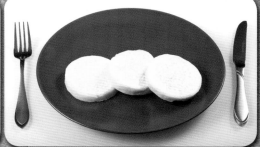

Weight: 182g

Index

D

E

F